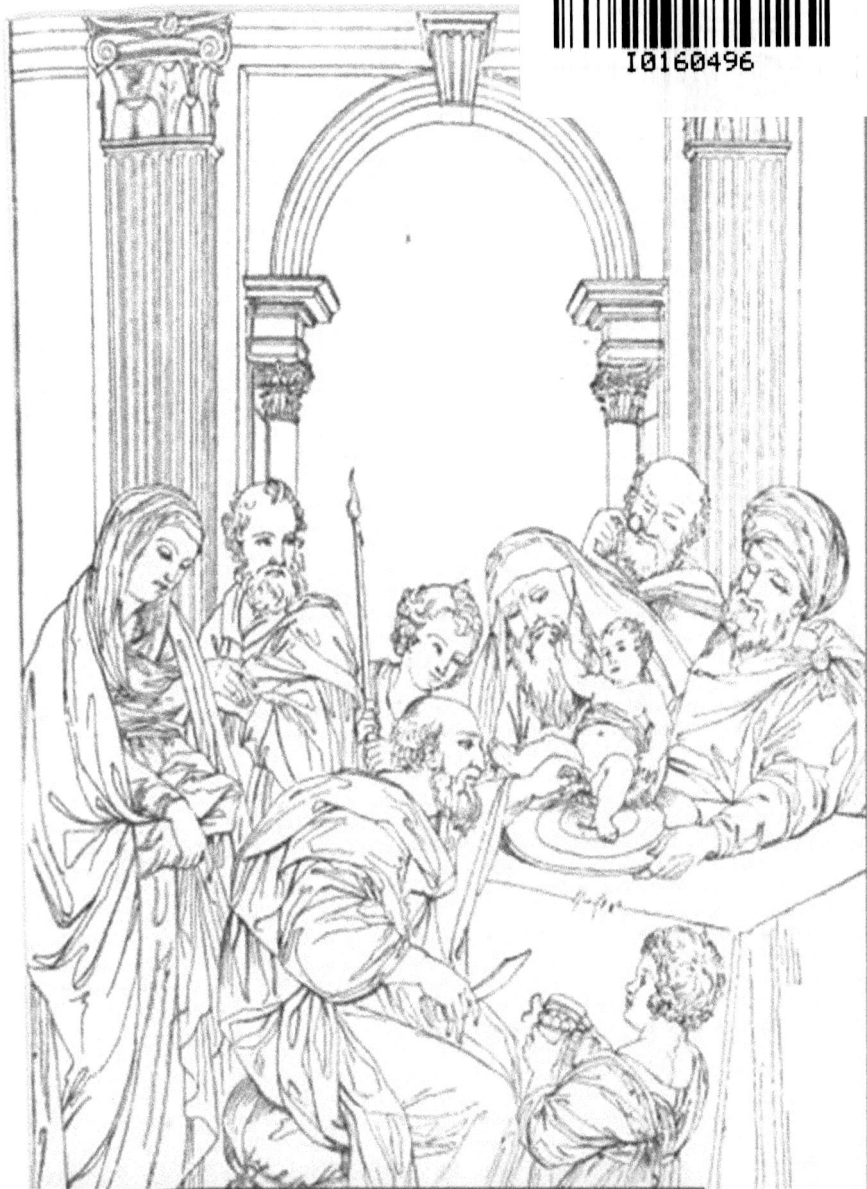

*History of circumcision, from
the earliest times to the present*

Peter Charles Remondino

Peter Charles Remondino

History of Circumcision from the Earliest Times to the Present—Moral and Physical Reasons for its Performance

Peter Charles Remondino, MD

With a history of eunuchism, hermaphrodism, and of the different operations practiced on the prepuce

Foreword by Allen Wyler, MD

Peter Charles Remondino

Originally published in 1891

Peter Remondino was a member of the American Medical Association, of the American Public Health Association, of the San Diego County Medical Society, of the State Board of Health of California, and of the Board of Health of the City of San Diego; Vice-President of California State Medical Society and of Southern California Medical Society, etc.

Publishers Note

For each copy of this book sold through the Stairway Press website, a donation of $5.00 will be made to Prostrate Cancer Foundation (www.pcf.org). If men were soft and cute like women are, then research for prostrate cancer would be funded just as well a breast cancer research.

STAIRWAY⬛PRESS

CAREFULLY SELECTED & EDITED BOOKS FOR DISCERNING AUDIENCES

www.StairwayPress.com

1500A East College Way #554
Mount Vernon, WA 98273

Front Illustration: HEBRAIC CIRCUMCISION
ISBN 978-0-9859942-9-7

HISTORY of CIRCUMCISION

FOREWORD

Circumcision commonly refers to the surgical removal of the foreskin from the penis. It may be surprising to some readers to learn that female circumcision is practiced in some African countries (the partial or total removal of a young girl's external genitalia) as a rite of passage into womanhood and marriage. Since the 1950s there has been increasing opposition to female circumcision arguing that the practice is detrimental to women's health and well-being and is considered a ritualized form of child abuse and a human rights violation, especially when no local anesthetic is used.

Male circumcision is highly cultural and religiously influenced. The act is prevalent in the Muslim world, parts of Southeast Asia, Africa, the United States and Oceania; it is relatively rare in Europe, Latin America, parts of Southern Africa, and most of Asia. The oldest documentary evidence for it comes from ancient Egypt. It is considered religious law in Judaism and established tradition in Islam.

In present day United States, the surgery is often performed in the newborn nursery using devices such as the Plastibell, or the Gomco or Mogen-style clamps. The foreskin is opened, inspected, and then separated from the glans. Anesthetic is commonly used. The clamp is placed carefully, detaching the foreskin. Complication rates are low and can include bleeding, infection and the removal of either too much or too little foreskin. Circumcision does not appear to negatively impact sexual function.

Circumcision may be indicated for both therapeutic and prophylactic reasons. Several studies of sexually transmitted disease show a marked decrease in spread of HIV and papillomavirus (HPV) from circumcised males both heterosexually and homosexually. For some males who suffer frequent urinary tract infections (UTI) circumcision may decrease the risk of recurrence. The explanation being that removal of the foreskin improves hygiene around the tip of the penis. Circumcision has a protective effect against the risks of penile cancer in men, and cervical cancer in the female sexual partners of heterosexual men.

In the United States, circumcision did not become common medical procedure until the late Victorian times. Circumcision was thought to prevent or cure an enormous and wide-ranging array of medical problems and social ills, including masturbation (considered by the Victorians to be an enormous problem), syphilis, epilepsy, hernia, headache, clubfoot, alcoholism and gout. By the turn of the century, in both American and Great Britain, infant circumcision was nearly universally recommended.

Neonatal circumcision is controversial because of the concept that all elective medical procedures must have consent of the patient. How can a neonate consent? On the other side of the issue, health care providers argue that parents should determine what is in the best interest of the infant or child who is incapable of providing informed consent.

Three parties are involved in the decision to

circumcise a minor: the minor, the parents (or Legal Authorized Representative) and the physician. The physician is bound under the ethical principles (set down in the Belmont Report) of beneficence (promoting well-being) and to do no harm. Those involved in the decision making must weigh what is in the best interest of the minor against the potential harms of the procedure.

Generally, circumcising a minor is not ethically controversial or legally questionable when there is a clear medical indication to justify it. The standard of care for conditions such as severe phimosis or a preputial tumor include circumcision.

However, circumcision is often considered for reasons other than to treat medical need. From the public health standpoint it can be a net benefit. Especially if the procedure is performed during the neonatal period when it is the most cost effective and carries the least risk of complications. Yet, critics argue that in the United States the number of circumcisions that would be needed to yield a public health benefit would be offset by the number of complications. There are counter arguments to this stance.

We operate under the assumption that parents have their child's best interests in mind when making these decisions and that they've been adequately inform of the benefits and risks of the procedure before consenting. However, many parents decide for or against circumcision before the child is born and for reasons other than health concerns.

So what is the right decision? Well, as an evidence-based practitioner, I tend to look to the experts for advice. In 2012, the American Academy of Pediatrics (AAP) stated that a systematic evaluation of the medical literature shows that the "preventive health benefits of elective circumcision of male newborns outweigh the risks of the procedure" and that the health benefits "are sufficient to justify access to this procedure for families choosing it and to warrant third-party payment for circumcision of male newborns," but "are not great enough to recommend routine circumcision for all male newborns." The AAP suggest that parents make the final decision after considering all appropriate information about the risks and benefits of the procedure. This is a shift in their position from their 1999 statement that stated the health benefits of the procedure outweigh the risks.

The AAP's 2012 position statement was also endorsed by the American College of Obstetricians and Gynecologists.

The AMA released 2011 policy statements that parents should be given the opportunity to make an informed choice regarding circumcision for their infant sons, and opposed attempts to make circumcision illegal.

The American Academy of Family Physicians (2007) recognizes the controversy surrounding circumcision and recommends that physicians "discuss the potential harms and benefits of circumcision with all parents or legal guardians considering this procedure for their newborn son."

The American Urological Association (2007) stated that neonatal circumcision has potential medical benefits and advantages as well as disadvantages and risks, stating that "while the results of studies in

History of Circumcision

African nations may not necessarily be extrapolated to men in the United States at risk for HIV infection, the American Urological Association recommends that circumcision should be presented as an option for health benefits. Circumcision should not be offered as the only strategy for HIV risk reduction. Other methods of HIV risk reduction, including safe sexual practices, should be emphasized."

—Allen Wyler, MD, 2012, Seattle, Washington

Peter Charles Remondino

PREFACE

In ancient Egypt the performance of circumcision was at one time limited to the priesthood, who, in addition to the cleanliness that this operation imparted to that class, added the shaving of the whole body as a means of further purification. The nobility, royalty, and the higher warrior class seem to have adopted circumcision as well, either as a hygienic precaution or as an aristocratic prerogative and insignia.

Among the Greeks we find a like practice, and we are told that in the times of Pythagoras the Greek philosophers were also circumcised, although we find no mention that the operation went beyond the intellectual class. In the United States, France, and in England, there is a class which also observe circumcision as a hygienic precaution, where, from my personal observation, I have found that circumcision is thoroughly practiced in every male member of many of the families of the class—this being the physician class.

In general conversation with physicians on this subject, it has really been surprising to see the large number who have had themselves circumcised, either through the advice of some college professor while attending lectures or as a result of their own subsequent convictions when engaged in actual practice and daily coming in contact both with the benefits that are to be derived in the way of a better physical, mental, and moral health, as well as with the many dangers and disadvantages that follow the uncircumcised—the latter being probably the most frequent incentive and determinator—as in many of

10

these latter examples the operation of circumcision, with its pains, annoyances, and possible and probable dangers, sink into the most trifling insignificance in comparison to some of the results that are daily observed as the tribute that is paid by the unlucky and unhappy wearer of a prepuce for the privilege of possessing such an appendage.

There is one thing that must be admitted concerning circumcision: this being that, among medical men or men of ordinary intelligence who have had the operation performed, instead of being dissatisfied, they have extended the advantages they have themselves received, by having those in their charge likewise operated upon. The practice is now much more prevalent than is supposed, as there are many Christian families where males are regularly circumcised soon after birth, who simply do so as a hygienic measure.

For the benefit of these, who may congratulate themselves upon the dangers and annoyances that they and their families have escaped, and for the benefit of those who would run into these dangers but for timely warning, this book has been especially written. To my professional brothers the book will prove a source of instruction and recreation, for, while it contains a lot of pathology regarding the moral and physical reasons why circumcision should be performed, which might be as undigestible as a mess of Boston brown bread and beans on a French stomach, I have endeavored to make that part of the book readable and interesting.

The operative chapter will be particularly useful and interesting to physicians, as I have there given a careful and impartial review of all the operative procedures—from the most simple to the most elaborate—besides paying more than particular attention to the subject of after-dressings. The part that relates to the natural history of man will interest all manner of people. I regret that the tabular statistics are not to be had, but in this regard we must use our best judgment from the material we have on hand; at any rate, I have tried to furnish a sufficiency of facts, so that, unless the reader is too overexacting, he will not find much difficulty in arriving at a conclusion on the subject.

—P. C. REMONDINO, M.D.

SAN DIEGO, CALIFORNIA, 1891.

Contents

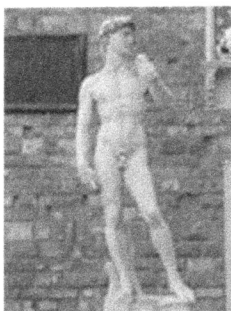

INTRODUCTION

This book is the amplification of a paper, the subject of which was *A Plea for Circumcision; or, the Dangers that Arise from the Prepuce,* which was read at the meeting of the Southern California Medical Society, at Pasadena, in December, 1889.

The material gathered for that paper was more than could be used in the ordinary limits of a society paper; it was gathered and ready for use, and this suggested its arrangement into book form. The subject of the paper was itself suggested by a long and personal observation of the changes made in man by circumcision. From the individual observation of cases, it was but natural to wish to enlarge the scope of our observation and comparison; this naturally led to a study of the physical characteristics of the only race that could practically be used for the purpose.

This race is the Jewish race. On carefully studying into the subject, I plainly saw that much of their longevity could consistently be ascribed to their more practical humanitarianism, in caring for their poor, their sick, as well as in their generous provision for their unfortunate aged people. The social fabric of the Jewish family is also more calculated to promote long life, as, strangely as it may seem, family veneration and family love and attachment are far more strong and practical among this people than among Christians, this sentiment not being even as strong in the Christian races as it is in the Chinese or Japanese.

It certainly forms as much of a part of the teachings of Christianity as it does of Judaism, Buddhism, or Confucianism, only Christians, as a mass, have practically forgotten it. The occupation followed by the Jews also in a certain degree favors longevity, and the influence on heredity induced by all these combined conditions goes for something. But it is not alone in the matter of simple longevity—although that implies considerable—that the Jewish race is found to be better situated. Actual observations show them to be exempt from many diseases which affect other races; so that it is not only that they recover more promptly, but that they are not, as a class, subjected to the loss of time by illness, or to the consequent sufferings due to illness or disease, in anything like or like ratio with other people.

There is also a less tendency to criminality, debauchery, and intemperance in the race; this, again, can in a measure be ascribed to their family influence, which even in our day has not lost that patriarchal influence which tinges the home or family life in the Old Testament. Crimes against the person or property committed by Jews are rare. They likewise do not figure in either police courts or penitentiary records; they are not inmates of our poor-houses, but, what is also singular, they are never accused of many silly crimes, such as indecent exposures, assaults on young girls; nor do they figure in any such exposures as the one recently made by the *Pall Mall Gazette.*

After allowing all that, which we can, in its fullest limit, to religion, family, or social habit, there is still a wide margin to be accounted for. This has naturally let the inquiry, followed in the course of this book, into a careful review of the Jewish people; into their religion and its character, its relation to other creeds, and to the world's history; into their many wanderings, and into the dispersion, and we have even been obliged to follow them into the midst of the people among whom they have become nationed, to try, if possible, to find the cause of this racial difference in health, resistance to disease, decay, and death.

It has been necessary, in following out the research, to give a condensed _résumé_ of the religious, political, and social condition of the Jewish commonwealth, which, although in a state of dispersion, still exists. I need offer no apology for the extended notice this has received in the course of the book.

We read with increasing interest either Hallam or May, Buckle or Guizot, through the spasmodic, halting, retrograding, advancing, erratic, aimless, and accidental phases that England has plowed through, from the days of goutless, simple, and chaste, but barbarian England of the Saxons, to the present civilized, enlightened, gouty, "Darkest England" of General Booth; and, after all is said and done, we are no wiser in any practical resulting good.

We simply know that the English people, so to speak, have, as it were, gone through the figures of

17

some social aspects, as if dancing the "Lancers," with its forward and back movements, gallop, etc., and have finally sat down, better dressed and better housed, but in an acquired state of moral and physical degeneration.

The Briton of Queen Victoria is not the Briton of Queen Boadicea, either morally or physically. On the other hand, the system of sociological tables adopted by Herbert Spencer would have but little to record for some six thousand years—either in religion, morals, or physique—as making any changes in the history of that simple people which, in the mountainous regions of Ur, in distant Armenia, started on its pilgrimage of life and racial existence; in one branch of the family— that of Ishmael—the changes to be recorded are so invisible that its descendants may really be said to live to-day as they lived then.

So that I do not feel that I need to apologize for the space I have given to this subject in the course of the book. The causes that make these racial distinctions should be of interest alike to the moralist, theologist, sociologist, and to the physician.

Ecclesiastical writers and moralists, as well as writers of fiction or dramatizers, can write on anything they please, and it is eagerly taken up and read by the people generally, either of high or low degree, alike; and somehow these people seem never to require an apology on the part of the author, for having attempted rapes, seductions, or even unavoidable fornication committed through the leaves of the story, or having it imaginably take place between acts on the stage.

But if the physician writes a book touching anything connected with the generative functions, and with the best intent and for the good of humanity, he is expected to make some prefatory apology. He is supposed to address a public who all of a sudden have become intensely moral and extremely sensitive in their modesty. Why things are thus I cannot explain. They are so, nevertheless. From the time that the celebrated Astruc wrote his treatise on female diseases, near the end of the seventeenth century—who felt compelled by the extreme modesty of the people in this particular—but who, outside of medicine, were about as virtuous as the average Tabby or Tom cats in the midnight hour—to write the chapter touching on nymphomania in Latin, so as not to shock the morbidly sensitive modesty of the French nobility, who then enjoyed *Le Droit de cuissage*—down through to Bienville, who wrote the first extended work on nymphomania, and Tissot, who first broached the subject and the danger of Onanism, all have felt that they must stop on the threshold and "apologize."

Tissot, however, seemed to possess a robust and a plain Hippocratic mind, and as he apologized he could not help but see the ridiculousness of so doing, as in the preface to his work we find the following: "Shall we remain silent on so important a subject?

By no means.

The sacred authors, the Fathers of the Church, who present their thoughts in living words, and ecclesiastical authors have not felt that silence was best. I have followed their example, and shall exclaim, with St. Augustine, 'If what I have written scandalizes any prudish persons, let them rather accuse the turpitude of their own thoughts than the words I have been obliged to use.'

Peter Charles Remondino

For my part, I think that people who can go to the theatre and enjoy "As in a Looking-Glass," and witness some of the satyrical or billy-goat traits of humanity so graphically exhibited in "La Tosca," with evident satisfaction; or attend the more robust plays of "Virginius" or of "Galba, the Gladiator," with all its suggestions of the Cæsarian section, and the lust and the fornications of an intensely animal Roman empress, without the destruction of their moral equilibrium or tending to induce in them a disposition to commit a rape on the first met—I think such people can be safely entrusted to read this book.

And as to the reading public, there are but few general readers who could honestly plead an ignorance of the "Decameron," Balzac, La Fontaine, "Heptameron," Crébillon *fils*, or of matter-of-fact Monsieur le Docteur Maitre Rabelais—works which, more or less, carry a moral instruction in every tale, which, like the tales of the "Malice of Women," in the unexpurged edition of the literal translation of the "Arabian Nights," contains much more of practical moral lessons, even if in the flowery and warm, spiced language of the Orient, than any supposed nastiness, on account of which they are classed among the prohibited.

To these, and the readers of Amelie Rives's books, or other intensely realistic literature, I need not imitate the warning of Ansonius, who warned his readers on the threshold of a part of his book to "stop and consider well their strength before proceeding with its lecture." Metaphorically speaking, the general theatre-going, or modern literature-reading public, can be considered pretty callous and morally bullet proof. I

20

shall therefore make no apology.

Some fault may, perhaps, be found with some of the occasional style of the book, or with some of the subjects used to illustrate a principle. To the extremely wise, good, and scientific, these illustrations were unnecessary; this need hardly be mentioned; and the passages which to some may prove objectionable were not intended for them, either with the expectation of delighting them or with the purpose of shocking them. These passages, they can easily avoid.

This book, however, was written that it might be read: not only read by the Solon, Socrates, Plato, or Seneca of the laity or the profession, but even by the billy-goated dispositioned, vulgar plebeian, who could no more be made to read cold, scientific, ungarnished facts than you can make an unwilling horse drink at the watering-trough.

Human weakness and perversity is silly, but it is sillier to ignore that it exists. So, for the sake of boring and driving a few solid facts into the otherwise undigesting and unthinking, as well as primarily obdurate understanding of the untutored plebeian, I ask the indulgence of the intelligent and broad-minded as well as the easily inducted reader.

Cleopatra was smuggled into Cæsar's presence in a roll of tapestry; the Greeks introduced their men into Troy by means of a wooden horse; and the discoverer of the broad Pacific Ocean made his escape from his importunate creditors disguised as a cask of merchandise. So, when we wish to accomplish an object, we must adopt appropriate means, even if they may apparently seem to have an entirely diametrically opposite object. The Athenian, Themistocles, when wishing to make the battle of Salamis decisive, was inspired with the idea of sending word to the Persian monarch that the Greeks were trying to escape, advising him to block the passage; this saved Greece.

There is a weird and ghostly but interesting tale connected with the Moslem conquest of Spain, of how Roderick, the last of the Gothic kings, when in trouble and worry, repaired to an old castle, in the secret recesses of which was a magic table whereon would pass in grim procession the different events of the future of Spain; as he gazed on the enchanted table he there saw his own ruin and his country's and nation's subjugation. Anatomy is generally called a dry study, but, like the enchanted brazen table in the ancient Gothic castle, it tells a no less weird or interesting tale of the past. Its revelations lighten up a long vista, through the thousands of years through which the human species has evolved from its earliest appearance on earth, gradually working up through the different evolutionary processes to what is to day supposed to be the acme of perfection as seen in the Indo-European and Semitic races of man.

Anatomy points to the rudiment—still lingering, now and then still appearing in some one man and without a trace in the next—of that climbing muscle which shows man in the past either nervously escaping up the trunk of a tree in his flight from many of the carnivorous animals with whom he was contemporary, or, as the shades of night were beginning to gather around him, we again see him by the aid of these muscles leisurely climbing up to some hospitable fork in the tree, where the robust habits of the age allowed him to find a comfortable resting-place;

protected from the dew of the night by the overhanging branches and from the prowling hyena by the height of the tree, he passed the night in security.

The now useless ear-muscles, as well as the equally useless series of muscles about the nose, also tell us of a movable, flapping ear capable of being turned in any direction to catch the sound of approaching danger, as well as of a movable and dilated nostril that scented danger from afar—the olfactory sense at one time having a different function and more essential to life than that of merely noting the differential aroma emitted by cigars or cups of Mocha or Java, and the ear being then used for some more useful purpose than having its tympanum tortured by Wagnerian discordant sounds.

Our ancestors might not have been a very handsome set, nor, judging from the Neanderthal skull, could they have had a very winning physiognomy, but they were a very hardy and self-reliant set of men. Nature—always careful that nothing should interfere with the procreative functions—had provided him with a sheath or prepuce, wherein he carried his procreative organ safely out of harm's way, in wild steeple-chases through thorny briars and bramble-brakes, or, when hardly pushed, and not able to climb quickly a tree of his own choice, he was by circumstances forced up the sides of some rough-barked or thorny tree. This leathery pouch also protected him from the many leeches, small aquatic lizards, or other animals that infested the marshes or rivers through which he had at times to wade or swim; or served as a protection from the bites of ants or other vermin when, tired, he rested on his haunches on some mossy bank or sand-hill.

Man has now no use for any of these necessaries of a long-past age—an age so remote that the speculations of Ernest Renan regarding the differences between the Semitic race of Shem and the idolatrous descendants of Ham, away off in the far mountains and valleys of Asia lying between the Mediterranean Sea and the Euphrates, seem more as if he were discussing an event of yesterday than something which is considered contemporary with our earlier history—and we find them disappearing, disuse gradually producing an obliteration of this tissue in some cases, and the modifying influence of evolution producing it in others; the climbing muscle, probably the oldest remnant and legacy that has descended from our long-haired and muscular ancestry, is the best example of disappearance caused by disuse, while the effectual disappearance of the prepuce in many cases shows that in that regard there exists a marked difference in the evolutionary march among different individuals.

There is a strange and unaccountable condition of things, however, connected with the prepuce that does not exist with the other vestiges of our arboreal or sylvan existence. Firstly, the other conditions have nothing that interferes with their disappearance; whereas the prepuce, by its mechanical construction and the expanding portions which it incloses, tends at times rather to its exaggerated development than to its disappearance.

Again, whereas the other vestiges have no injury that they inflict by their presence, or danger that they cause their possessors to run, the prepuce is from time of birth a source of annoyance, danger, suffering, and death. Then, again, the other conditions are not more developed at birth; whereas the prepuce seems, in our pre-natal life, to have an unusual and unseen-for-use existence, being in bulk out of all proportion to the organ it is intended to cover. Speculation as to its existence is as unprolific of results as any we may indulge in regarding the nature, object, or uses of that other evolutionary appendage, the appendix vermiformis, the recollection of whose existence always adds an extra flavor to tomatoes, figs, or any other small-seeded fruits.

We may well exclaim, as we behold this appendage to man—now of no use in health and of the most doubtful assistance to the very organ it was intended to protect, when that organ, through its iniquitous tastes, has got itself into trouble, and, Job-like, is lying repentant and sick in its many wrappings of lint, with perhaps its companions in crime imprisoned in a suspensory bandage—what is this prepuce?

Whence, why, where, and whither?

At times, Nature, as if impatient of the slow march of gradual evolution, and exasperated at this persistent and useless as well as dangerous relic of a far-distant prehistoric age, takes things in her own hands and induces a sloughing to take place, which rids it of its annoyance. In the far-off land of Ur, among the mountainous regions of Kurdistan, something over six thousand years ago, the fathers of the Hebrew race, inspired by a wisdom that could be nothing less than of divine origin, forestalled the process of evolution by establishing the rite of circumcision. Whether this has been beneficial or injurious to the race will be, in a measure, the object of the discussion in this book.

One object of this book is to furnish my professional brothers with some embodied facts that they may use in convincing the laity in many cases where they themselves are convinced that circumcision is absolutely necessary; but, having nothing in their text-books to back up their opinion with, their explanations are too apt to pass for their mere unfounded personal view of the matter.

If the patient, or the parents of the patient, ask the physician for his authority, he is at a loss, as there is nothing that deals with the subject in any extended manner; so that this book has been written in as plain English as the subject-matter could possibly allow, so that non-professionals could easily read and understand it.

I have often felt the need of such a work; people can understand emergency or accident surgery, military surgery, or reparative surgery, but such a thing as surgery to remedy a seemingly medical disease, or what might be called the preventive practice of surgery, is something they cannot understand. First, and not the least, among the incentives to skepticism on this subject is the unwelcome fact of a surgical operation, which, no matter how trivial it may seem to the surgeon, is a matter of considerable magnitude to the patient, his parents, or friends; there are risks, pain, worry, annoyances, and expenses to be undergone—considerations which, either singly or unitedly, often lead one to reason against the operation, even when otherwise convinced of its need or utility.

The hardest to convince are those, however, who insist on having a four-and-a-half-foot-gauge fact driven through their two-foot-gated understanding, without it ever occurring to them that the gate, and not the fact, is the faulty article, Some of these gentry are very unconvincible. They at times remind one of that description given by Carlyle in regard to one of the Georges, who found himself, when Prince of Wales, leading an army in Flanders, and actually engaged in a battle. His Royal Highness was on foot, and was seen standing facing the enemy, with outstretched legs, like a Colossus of Rhodes, impassive and stolid—the very impersonification of Dutch courage and aggressiveness.

There he stood, unconscious whether he was at the head of an army or single attendant; he might be overridden and annihilated, overturned and expunged, but there he would most assuredly stand and fall, if need be; overwhelming squadrons, by their impetus and weight, might ride him down and crush him; but one thing was most certain, this certain fact being that he never could be made to retreat or advance, as no impression from front or rear could convince him of the necessity of either.

Then, there is our statistical friend, who cannot discriminate between the exception and the rule by any common-sense deductions. He must have all the authentic, carefully-compiled statistics before he can allow himself to form any opinion. As long as there is the smallest fraction of a decimal unaccounted for in a mathematical way, this individual is inconvincible. These men pride themselves upon being methodically exact; they express their willingness to be convinced if you can present acceptable proofs; but, trying to present simple rational proofs to these individuals is considerably like presenting a meal of boiled pork and cabbage to a confirmed and hypochondriacal dyspeptic—it only increases their mental dyspepsia.

Had Columbus waited to discover America, or had Galileo waited to proclaim the motion of the earth, until authorized to a serious consideration of the matter by properly-tabled statistics, they would have waited a long, long time; and, it may be added, the inconveniences that attend the proving of a negative will so interfere with the proper arrangement of statistical matter which relates to the prepuce and circumcision that, before such tables could be satisfactorily and convincingly constructed, time and the evolutionary processes that follow it will bid fair to completely remove this debatable appendage from man. It may be at a very far-distant period that this evolutionary preputial extinction will take place— probably contemporary with the existence of Bulwer's "Coming Race,"—but not at a too remote period for the proper and satisfactory tabulation of the statistics.

The ideas of the etiology and pathological processes through which we journey—from a condition of health and good feeling to one of disease, miserable feeling, and death—as described in, or rather as they control the sentiment and policy of, this work, are such as have been followed by Hutchinson, Fothergill, Beale, Black, Albutt, and Richardson, so that if I have totally ignored the old conventional systems, with their hide-bound classification of diseases to control the etiology, I have not done so without some reliable authority.

In studying the etiology of diseases we have, as a

rule, been content to accept the disease when fully formed and properly labeled, being apparently satisfied with beginning our investigation not at the initial point of departure from health, but at some distant point from this, at the point where this departure has elaborated itself, on favorable ground, into a tangible general or local disease. As truthfully observed by T. Clifford Albutt: "The philosophic inquirer is not satisfied to know that a person is suffering, for example, from a cancer. He desires to know why he is so suffering—that is, what are the processes which necessarily precede or follow it. He wishes to include this phenomena, now isolated, in a series of which it must necessarily be but a member, to trace the period of which it must be but a phase. He believes that diseased processes have their evolution and the laws of it, as have other natural processes, and he believes that these are fixed and knowable."

To do this, the physician must travel beyond the beaten path of etiology as found in our textbooks. He must follow Hutchinson in the train of reasoning that elucidates the pre-cancerous stage of cancer, or tread in the path followed by Sir Lionel Beale, in finding that the cause of disease depends on a blood change and the developmental defect, or the tendency or inherent weakness of the affected part or organ; to fully appreciate the inherent etiological factors that reside in man, and which constitute the tendency to disease or premature decay and death, we must also be able to follow Canstatt, Day, Rostan, Charcot, Rush, Cheyne, Humphry, or Reveille-Parise into the study of the different conditions which, though normal, are nevertheless factors of a slow or a long life.

We must also be able to appreciate fully the value of that interdependence of each part of our organism, which often, owing to a want of equilibrium of strength and resistance in some part when compared to the rest, causes the whole to give way, just as a flaw in a levee will cause the whole of the solidly-constructed mass to give way, or a demoralized regiment may entail the utter rout of an army.

As described by George Murray Humphry, in his instructive work on "Old Age," at page 11:

> The first requisite for longevity must clearly be an inherent or inborn quality of endurance, of steady, persistent nutritive force, which includes reparative force and resistance to disturbing agencies, and a good proportion or balance between the several organs. Each organ must be sound in itself, and its strength must have a due relation to the strength of the other organs. If the heart and the digestive system be disproportionately strong, they will overload and oppress the other organs, one of which will soon give way; and, as the strength of the human body, like that of a chain, is to be measured by its weaker link, one disproportionately feeble organ endangers or destroys the whole. The second requisite is freedom from exposure to the various casualties, indiscretions, and other causes of disease to which illness and early death are so much due.

In following out our study of diseases, we have been too closely narrowed down by the old symptomatic story of disease; we have too much treated surface symptoms, and neglected to study the man and his surroundings as a whole; we have overlooked the fact that there exists a geographical fatalism in a physical sense as well as the existence of the influence of that climatic fatalism so well described by Alfred Haviland, and the presence of a fatalism of individual constitution as well, which is either inherited or acquired.

The idea that Charcot elaborates, that, as the year passes successively through the hot and the cold, through the dry and the wet season, with advancing age the human body undergoes like changes, and diseases assume certain characteristics, are also points that are overlooked; and nowhere is this latter view seen to be more neglected than in the relations the prepuce bears to infancy, prime and old age, as will be more fully explained in the chapters in this book which treat of cancer and gangrene. Admitting that Haviland has exaggerated the influence of climate as an etiological factor in its specific influence in producing certain diseases; or that M. Taine claims more than he should for his "Thèorie des Milieux," or influence of surroundings; or that Hutchinson has drawn the hereditary and pedigreeal fatherhood of disease too finely; it must also be admitted that the solid, tangible truths upon which these authors have founded their premises are plainly visible to the most skeptical; the architectural details of the superstructure may be defective, but the foundation is permanent.

From the above outline it will be easier for the reader to follow out the reasons, or the whys or wherefores, of the views expressed on medicine in the course of the book; and, although I do not wish to enter the medical field like a Peter the Hermit on a new crusade, to lure thousands into the hands of the circumcisers, nor, as a new Mohammed, promise the eternal bliss and glory of the seventh heaven to all the circumcised, I ask of my professional brothers a calm and unprejudiced perusal of the tangible and authentic facts that I have honestly gathered and conscientiously commented upon from my field of vision, which will be plainly presented in the following pages. I simply have given the facts and my impressions: the reader is at liberty to draw his own conclusions.

If I have been too tedious in the multiplication of incidents in support of certain views, I must remind the reader that the verdict goes to him who has the preponderance of testimony, and that many a lawsuit is lost from the neglect, on the part of the loser, to secure all the available testimony. Having brought the subject of circumcision before the bar of public opinion, as well as that of my professional brother, I would but illy do justice to the subject at the bar, or to myself, not to properly present the case; as it was remarked by Napoleon, "God is on the side of the heaviest artillery," and he who loses a battle for want of guns should not rail at Providence if, having them on hand, he has neglected to bring them into action.

The reasons for the existence of the book will become self-evident as the reader labors through the medical part of the work. Our textbooks are, as a class, even those on diseases of children as a specialty, singularly and unpardonably silent and deficient on the subject of either the prepuce and the diseases to which it leads, or circumcision; and even our surgical works are not sufficiently explicit, as they deal more with the developed disease and the operative measures for its removal than on any preventive surgery or medicine. Our works on medicine are equally silent, and, although from a perusal of the latter part of the book the prepuce and circumcision will be seen to have considerable bearing on the production and nature of phthisis, this subject would, owing to our strabismic way of studying medicine, look most singularly out of place in a work devoted to diseases of the lungs or throat. Owing to this poverty of literature on the subject, and that the library of the average practitioner could therefore not furnish all the data relating to it that the profession have in their possession, a book of this nature will furnish them the required material whereupon to form the basis of an opinion on the subject.

To argue that the prepuce is not such a deadly appendage because so many escape alive and well who are uncircumcised, would be as logical as to assume that Lee's chief of artillery neglected to properly place his guns on the heights back of Fredericksburg. He had asserted, the night before the battle, that not a chicken could live on the intervening plateau between the heights and the town. On the next day, when these guns opened their fire, the Federals were unable to reach the heights, while many men were for hours in the iron hail-sweeping discharges of that artillery that mowed them down by whole ranks, and yet the majority escaped alive. We take the middle ground, and, while admitting that many escape alive with a prepuce, claim that more are crippled than are visibly seen, as, like Bret Harte's "Heathen Chinee," the ways of the prepuce are dark and mysterious as well as peculiar.

A discussion of the relative merits of religious creeds, when considered in relation to health, has been, from the nature of the subject of the book, unavoidable. Modern Christianity but very imperfectly explains why this rite was either neglected or abolished. Frequent reference is made to what Saint Paul said and did, but, as Saint Paul was not one of the Disciples, it is inexplicable wherefrom he received his authority in this matter, seeing that the Disciples themselves had no new views on the subject.

To the student who prefers to study his subject from all its aspects, the question naturally arises, "Where, when, and why came the authority that abolished this rite?" There is one probable explanation, this being that Paul, who was the real promulgator of Gentile Christianity, had to establish his creed among an uncircumcised race; although, as we shall see, devotees have not scrupled to sacrifice their virility in the hope of being more acceptable to God and to be better able to observe His commandments, and others, in their blind bigotry, have not objected to sitting naked on sand-hills, with a six-inch iron ring passed through the prepuce, it is very evident that the Apostle Paul's good sense showed him the uselessness of attempting to found the new creed, and at the same time hold on to the truly distinctive marking of Judaism among Gentiles, the Hebrew race being those among whom he found the least converts, as even the Disciples and Apostles in Palestine disagreed with him. In the words of Dr. I. M. Wise, it was impossible for the Palestine Apostles, or their flock, either to acknowledge Paul as one of their own set or submit to his teaching; for they obeyed the Law and he abolished it; they were sent to the house of Israel only, and Paul sought the Gentiles with the message that the Covenant and the Law were at an end; they had one gospel story and he another; they prophesied the speedy return of the Master and a restoration of the throne of David in the kingdom of heaven, and he prophesied the end of the world and the last day of judgment to be at hand; they forbade their converts to eat of unclean food, and especially of the sacrificial meats of the Pagans, and he made light of both, as well as of the Sabbath and circumcision.

In the attempted reconciliation that subsequently took place in Jerusalem at the house of James, the Jacob of Kaphersamia of the Talmud, Paul was charged by the synod of Jewish Christians "with disregarding the Law, forsaking the teachings of Moses, and attempting to abolish circumcision." He was bid to recant and undergo humiliation with four other Nazarenes, that it might be known that he walked orderly and observed the Law; Paul submitted to all that was demanded.

This, in short, with the exception of the sayings of Paul on the subject, which are all secondary considerations, is really all that there is relating to the abolishment of circumcision by the Christians.

The real Disciples and Apostles believed in Jesus with as much fervor as Paul, but it is singular that

35

they who were with the Master should always have insisted on the observance of the Law, while Paul as energetically insisted on its abolishment.

From these premises, I have seen fit to inquire into the relative merits of the three religions practiced by what we call the civilized nations, as they affect man morally, physically, and mentally. I have given the facts, my impressions, and reasons for being so impressed; from these, the reader can easily see that religion has more to do with man's temporal existence than is generally believed; its discussion is not, therefore, out of place in this book.

Repetitions in the course of the work have been unavoidable. This is not a novel nor a work of fiction, and wherever the want of repetition would have been an injury, either to the proper representation of a fact or a principle, the repetition has not been avoided. In describing the operations, I had desired to avoid any too numerous descriptions, as that is confusing, but have thought it best to give a number, as the reader will thereby obtain the views of the different operators, the mode of the operation often being an index to the view of the operator in regard to the needs or utility of a prepuce.

In the general plan of the work, I have adopted the idea and the historical relation carried out by Bergmann, of Strasburg, who included all the mutilations practiced on the genitals while discussing the subject of circumcision, they being, in the originality of performance, somewhat intimately connected; this also tends to make the subject more interesting as a contribution to the natural history of man—something in which all intelligent persons are more or less interested.

—P. C. REMONDINO, M.D.
SAN DIEGO, CALIFORNIA.

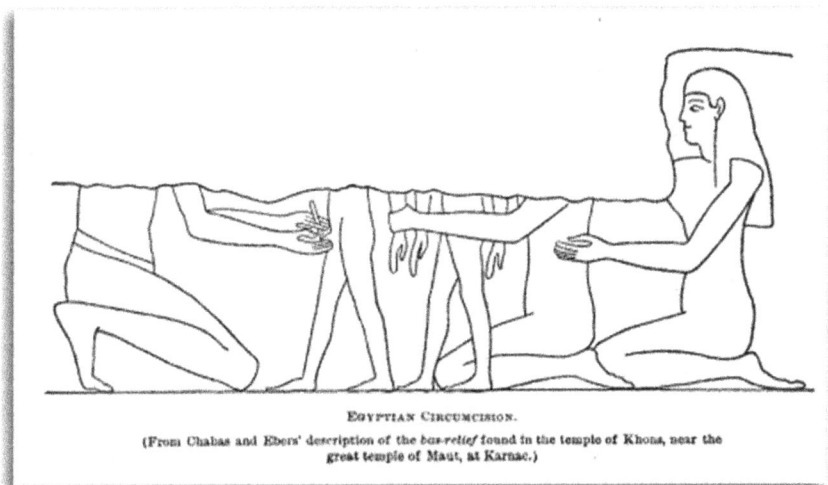

EGYPTIAN CIRCUMCISION.

(From Chabas and Ebers' description of the *bas-relief* found in the temple of Khons, near the great temple of Maut, at Karnac.)

EGYPTIAN CIRCUMCISION

From Chabas and Ebers' description of the bas-relief found in the temple of Khons, near the great temple of Maut, at Karnac.

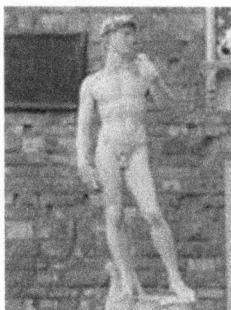

CHAPTER I—ANTIQUITY OF CIRCUMCISION

If the ceremonials of the Catholic Church or the High Church Episcopalians carry us back into the depths of antiquity, or, as remarked by Frothingham, that the ceremonies of St. Peter, at Rome, carried him back to the mysteries of Eulesis, to the sacrificial rites of ancient Phoenicia, to what misty antiquity does not the contemplation of the rite of circumcision take us?

The Alexandrian library, with its vast collection of precious records, could probably have furnished us some information as to its origin and antiquity; but Moslem fanaticism, with its belief in the all-sufficiency and infallibility of the Koran, was the destruction of that wonderful repository.

We must now depend wholly on the relation of the Old Testament or on what has since been written by the Greek and Italian historians as to its origin and practices. The Egyptian monuments and their hyeroglyphics give us no information on the subject further back than the reign of Rameses II; while the oft-quoted Herodotus wrote some fourteen centuries after the Old Testament relation, and Strabo and

Diodorus some nineteen centuries after the same chronicler.

We have, therefore, in their chronological order, first, the relation of the Bible; then the Egyptian monuments and their revelations; and, thirdly, the information gathered by Pythagoras, Herodotus, and other philosophers and historians. To these three sources we may add the misty mixture of tradition and mythological events, whose beginnings as to period of time are indefinite. These are the sources from which we are to determine the origin and antiquity as well as the character of the rite.

Voltaire found in the subject of circumcision one that he could not satisfactorily make enter into his peculiar system of general philosophy. For some reason, he did not wish that the Israelites should have the credit of its introduction; were he to have admitted that, he would have had to explain away the divine origin of the rite—something that the Hebrew has tenaciously held for over thirty-seven centuries.

Voltaire thought it would simplify the subject by making it originate with the Egyptians, from whom the Hebrews were to borrow it. To do this he adopted the relation of Herodotus on the subject. His treatment of the Jewish race, however, brought out a strong antagonism from those people to his attacks, and in a volume entitled *Letters of Certain Jews to Monsieur Voltaire*—being a series of criticisms on his aspersions on the race and on the writings of the Old Testament (written by a number of Portuguese, German, and Polish Jews then residing in Holland[1]—they proved

---

[1] *Letters of Certain Jews to Monsieur Voltaire, Containing an*

conclusively that the Phoenicians had borrowed the rite from the Israelites, as they (the Phoenicians) had practiced the rite on the newborn, whereas, had they followed the Egyptian rite, they would have only circumcised the child after its having passed its thirteenth year—these being the distinctive differences between the Jewish and Egyptian rites.

Luckily, in the small temple of Khons, which formed an annex to the greater temple of Maut, at Karnac, there was found a *bas-relief*, partly perfect, which goes far toward giving light on the subject of Egyptian circumcision.

The upper part of the sculpture was so defaced that the upper portions of four of the five figures were destroyed, but the lower portions were so perfect in every detail as to furnish a full history of the age of the candidates for the rite and the manner of its performance. It is further interesting from the fact that it establishes also the time during which the rite was so performed. M. Chabas and Dr. Ebers argue, from the founder of the temple having been Rameses II, that the sculpture refers to the circumcision of two of his children. The knife appears to be a stone implement, and the operator kneels in front of the child, who is standing, while a matron supports him in a kneeling posture, and she holds his hands from behind him.[2] In this *bas-relief* we can see the great difference that existed between the two forms of the operation, that of

---

Apology for their own People. Pages 451-476. Translated by Dr. Lefann. Philadelphia, 1848.

[2] *Circoncision chez les Egyptiens.* Brochure by F. Chabas. Paris, 1861.

the Hebrews being performed, as a rule, on the eighth day after birth, while in *the bas-relief* they are ten or twelve years old.

Although tradition and mythology veil past events in more or less obscurity, they do, in regard to circumcision, furnish considerable explanatory light on matters which would be otherwise hard to reconcile. Circumcision has been performed by the Chippeways in the Upper Mississippi, and its modifications were performed among the Mexicans, Central Americans, and some South American tribes of Indians, as well as among many of the natives dwelling among the islands of the Pacific Archipelago. There is a tradition, mentioned by Donnelly in connection with the sunken continent of Atlantis, that Ouranos, one of the Atlantean kings, ordered his whole army to be circumcised that they might escape a fatal scourge then decimating the people to their westward.[3] This tradition tells us that the hygienic benefits of circumcision were recognized antediluvian facts, as it also points out the way by which circumcision traveled westward across to the Western World.

As Donnelly has pointed out, many of the Americans possessed not only traditions, habits, and customs that must have come from the Old World, but the similarity of many words and their meaning that exists between some of the American languages and those of the indigenous inhabitants that have still their remains in spots on the southwestern shores of Europe—the ancient Armorica whose colony in Wales

---

[3] *Atlantis.* By Ignatius Donnelly. Page 472.

still retains its ancient words—leaves no room for doubt that at one time a landed highway existed between the two worlds.

The Mandans, on the Upper Missouri, have many words of undoubted Armorican origin in their vocabulary,[4] just as the Chiapenec, of Central America, contains its principal words denotive of deity, family relations, and many conditions of life that are identically the same as in the Hebrew,[5] the name of father, son, daughter, God, king, and rich being essentially the same in the two languages. It must have been more than a passing coincidence that gives the Mandans some of their most expressive words from the Welsh, or that gave to Central America many cities bearing analogous names with the cities of Armenia.[6] Canadian names of localities, as well as those of the Mississippi Valley, denote the French origin of their pioneers, as well as the names of Upper California denote the nationality and creed of its first settlers. So that there is nothing strange in asserting that American civilization and many of the customs as found in the fifteenth century by the early Spanish discoverers were nothing more than the remains of ancient and modified Phoenician civilization, among which figured circumcision.

Dr. A. B. Arnold, of Baltimore, argues that, with the present state of our anthropological knowledge and the material that research has been able to furnish, we need no longer be surprised to find customs, laws, and

---

[4] *Ibid.*, page 115.
[5] *Ibid.*, page 234.
[6] *Ibid.*, page 178.

morals, among nations living in regions of the world widely apart from each other, which betray an identity of origin and development, and that beliefs and institutions, whether wise or aberrant, grow up under apparently dissimilar circumstances, circumcision forming no exception.[7]

Dr. Arnold leaves too much to chance. It is hardly likely that the similarity that existed between the architecture of the Phoenicians and the Central Americans, as evinced in their arches; in the beginning of the century on the 26th of February; the advancement and interest taken in astronomical science; the coexistence of pyramids in Egypt and Central America; that five Armenian cities should have their namesakes in Central America, should all be a matter of accident.

The historiographer of the Canary Islands, M. Benshalet, considers that those islands once formed a part of the great continent to its west; this has been verified by the discovery of many sculptured symbols, similar in the Canaries and on the shores of Lake Superior, as well as by the discovery of a mummy in the Canaries with sandals whose exact counterparts were found in Central America.[8] A compound word used to signify the Great Spirit being found identical in the Welsh and Mandan languages, each requiring five distinct sounds to pronounce, words as intricate as the passwords of secret societies, can hardly be said to

---

[7] *Circumcision*. A. B. Arnold. *New York Med. Record*, Feb. 13, 1886.

[8] *Atlantis*, page 178.

be the result of chance.[9]

There must, at some remote period, have existed some communication between the ancestors of these Missouri Mandans and the shores of ancient Armorica; the ancestors of these Mandans may have then been living farther to the east; they even may have then been a tribe of since lost Atlantis; but the analogy, not only in regard to the word just mentioned—*Maho-peneta*, of the Welsh and Mandan—but in the similarity of the pronouns of both languages, and the existence of the idea of the counterpart of the sacred white bull of the Egyptians being found among the Dakotas, or Sioux, all point to the fact that these people, in common with the rest of the Americans, originally came from the East; from whence came their languages, manners, customs, rites, and what civilization they possessed, among which circumcision has, through the mist of centuries, held its own in some shape or other.

That some terrible catastrophe occurred to divide the hemispheres is evident; the Western World remaining stationary in its civilization and retaining the customs and rites of the times as evidence of their origin. With this view of the case, the existence of circumcision as found among the inhabitants of the West can easily be traced to its origin among the hills of Chaldea.

The ancient traditions and mythological relations of the Egyptians in regard to the great nation to the West are amply verified by the deep-sea soundings of

---

[9] This word is, in the Mandan, *Maho-peneta*; in the Welsh, *Mawr-penæthir*. *Atlantis*, page 115.

the "Challenger," the "Dolphin," and the "Gazelle," which plainly indicate the presence of a submarine plateau that once formed the continent of Atlantis, whose only visible evidence above the waves of the boisterous Atlantic is the Azores and the remains of Phoenician civilization among the Americans. Professor Worman, of Brooklyn, scouts the idea that circumcision was ever connected in any way or that it originated in any of the rites connected with phallic worship.[10]

Bergmann, [11] of Strasburg, however, not only claims circumcision to be a direct result of phallic worship, but looks upon the rite as something that has been reached by what may be termed a gradual evolutionary process of manners, customs, and society, from the time of what is termed the hero-warrior period of traditional history, when war and the clashing of shields and sword or spear were the main delights and occupations of man. It is strange to note what difference must have existed between these hero-warriors in regard to their ideas of manliness; some were brutal and fiendish, whilst others were magnanimous.

McPherson, the historiographer of early Britain, cannot help but contrast the superior manliness of the heroes of Ossian in his graphic description of the

---

[10] *Cyclopedia of Biblical, Theological, and Ecclesiastical Literature*, vol. viii, page 58. Article, Phallus.

[11] *Origine, Signification et Histoire, de la Castration, de l'eunuchism, et la circoncision.* Par. F. Bergmann. Published in the *Archivio per le Traditione Populaire*, 1883.

ancient Caledonians, when compared to the brutality of Homer's Greek heroes. The traditions upon which Bergmann undertakes to found the origin of the rite of circumcision are all connected with the inhuman and brutish passions that animated our barbarous ancestry.

The first incident given is the Egyptian traditional tragedy, which was, in all probability, the initial point of that phallic worship which, with increasing debauchery, assisted in the final demoralization of Rome and Greece, after its introduction into those countries.

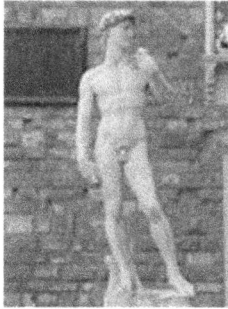

CHAPTER II—THEORIES AS TO THE ORIGIN OF CIRCUMCISION

We are told that in battle man looked upon the vanquished as unfit to bear the name of man, looking upon the weakness or want of skill which contributed to their defeat as something effeminate. The victor then proceeded by a very summary and effective mode, done in the most primitive and expeditious manner, to render his victim as much like a female as possible to all outward appearances; this was accomplished by a removal at one sweep of *all* the organs of eneration, the phallus being generally retained as a trophy—a practice which was also carried into effect with dead enemies, to show that the victor had vanquished *men*.

It has been the practice from time immemorial for a victor to carry off some portion of the body of his victim or defeated enemy, as a mark or testimony of his prowess; it was either a hand, head or scalp, lower jaw, or finger. The carrying off of the phallus or virile member was considered the most conclusive proof of the nature of the vanquished, and, as it established the sex, it conferred a greater title to bravery and skill than a mere collection of hands or scalps, which would not denote the sex.

In conformity with this custom, we find that Osiris, when he returned to Egypt and found that Typhon had fomented dissension in his absence, being vanquished by the latter in the conflict that followed, was dismembered and cut into pieces, the followers of Typhon each securing a piece and Typhon himself securing the phallus or generative member.

Isis, the spouse of Osiris, seems in turn to have secured the control of government, and, having secured all the pieces of the dissected Osiris except the phallus—Typhon having fled with that, and, according to some traditions, having thrown it into the sea—Isis ordered that statues should be constructed, each to contain a piece of the unfortunate Osiris, who should thereafter be worshiped as a god, and that the priesthood should choose from among the animals some one kind which should thereafter be considered sacred.

The phallus which was missing was ordered special worship, with more marked solemnities and mysteries; from this originated the phallic worship and the sacredness of the white bull, Apis, among the Egyptians, which was chosen to represent Osiris.

By gradual evolution and the progress of society, the cultivation of the ground and the need of menials, warriors found some other use for their prisoners taken in strife besides merely cutting off the phallus as a trophy; these prisoners began to have some intrinsic value. From this a change came about; the warrior instinct, however, still claimed that the vanquished, even if a slave, should still convey or carry some sign of servitude.

The original idea of the ablation of the phallus was to emasculate the victim; investigation developed the idea that the same object could be accomplished by castration, an operation which also finally reached a tolerable state of perfection through different stages of evolution, it first being performed by a complete removal of the whole scrotum and contents. This operation, with the ignorance of the times in regard to stopping hæmorrhage, was, however, accompanied by a large mortality, and it finally evolved into the simple removal of the gland, or its obliteration by pressure or violence. Bergmann conveys the idea that circumcision was at one time the indestructible marking and the distinctive feature of the slave, the mind of the period not being able to emancipate itself from the idea that the genitals must in some manner be mutilated, not being able to conceive any other degrading mark of manhood which barbarians felt they must inflict on slaves.

The generally accepted idea in regard to the physical mutilation of captives taken in war, or that some token from the body of the vanquished must be carried off by the victor, has not only the support of tradition and monumental sculptured evidence, but its practice is still in vogue among many races.

Among the ancient Scythians, only the warriors who returned from the battle or foray with the heads of the enemy were entitled to a share in the spoils.

Among the modern Berbers it is still a practice for a young man, on proposing marriage, to exhibit to his prospective father-in-law the virile members of all the enemies he has overcome, as evidence of his manhood and right to the title of warrior.

The Abyssinians and some of the negro tribes on the Guinea coast still follow the custom of securing the phallus of a fallen foe. However barbarous this practice may seem, its actual performance is only secondary, the primary motive being that the warrior wished to prove that he had been there, engaged in actual strife, and that his enemy had been overcome. The writer remembers that, after one of the battles in the West during the late war, many letters arrived in his locality with pieces of the garments or locks of the hair of the unfortunate Confederate general, Zollikoffer, who had been slain in the battle; a disposition in the warrior, seemingly still existing, such as animated the old Egyptians.

On an old Egyptian monument—that of Osymandyas—Diodorus noticed a mural sculpture, a *bas-relief* representing prisoners of war, either in chains or bound with cords, being registered by a royal scribe preparatory to losing either the right hand or the phallus, a pile of which is visible in one corner of the foreground; from this sculpture we learn that the practice was not only an individual performance, but that it was a national usage among the Egyptians as well, who subjected, at times, their vanquished foes to its ordeal in a wholesale but business-like manner.

Bergmann argues that the Israelites were given to like practices, and cites the incident wherein David brought two hundred prepuces—as evidence of his having slaughtered that number of Philistines—to Saul, as a mark of his being worthy to be his son-in-law. He argues that, whereas many have made that Old

Testament passage to read "two hundred prepuces," it should have read "two hundred virile members" which David and his companions had cut off from the Philistines, the word *orloth* meaning the virile member, and not the prepuce.

That Israelitish circumcision could have originated from either phallic worship or any of the hero-warrior usages is untenable as a proposition, as regards the living prisoners, and is contrary to the monotheistic idea which ruled Israel, or to the benign nature of their God. The strict opposition of the religion of Judaism to any other mutilation except that of the covenant is also antagonistic to the views advanced by Bergmann, as it is well known that even emasculated animals were considered imperfect and unclean, and therefore unfit to be received or offered as a sacrifice to their deity.

No emasculated man was allowed to enter the priesthood or assist at sacrifices. The whole idea of Judaism being opposed to such mutilations, their observance of circumcision and its performance can in no way have developed from either phallic or other warlike rites or usages; but we must accept its origin as a purely religious rite—a covenant of the most rigid observance, coincident in its inception with the formation of the Hebraic creed in the hills of Chaldea.

What Herodotus or Pythagoras may have written concerning the practice among the Egyptians was written, as already remarked, some nine centuries after Moses had recorded his laws; Moses himself having come some centuries after Abraham. Herodotus is quoted as representing that the Phoenicians borrowed the practice from the Egyptians, in support of the theory that Egypt was the central nucleus from whence the practice started, and not that it traveled toward Egypt from Phoenicia.

The difference in the ages, already mentioned, at which the rite was practiced—that of Phoenicia and Israel being at one time identical—shows that the testimony of Herodotus in this one particular was the result of faulty judgment, as we find the people who have borrowed the practice from the Egyptians, as well as their descendants, closely follow their practice in regard to the age at which the operation should be performed. Another evidence of the strictly religious nature of the rite, as far as the Hebrews are concerned, lies in the fact that, with all their skill in surgery and medical sciences—they being at one time the only intelligent exponents of our science—they never made any alteration or improvement in the manner of performing the operation.

It is evident that even Maimonides, a celebrated Jewish physician of the twelfth century, who furnished some rules in regard to the operation, was held under some constraint by the religious aspect of the rite. As a summary of this part of the subject, it may be stated that the Old Testament furnished the only reliable and authentic relation prior to Pythagoras and Herodotus. From its evidence, Abraham was the first to perform the operation, which he seems to have performed on himself, his son, and servants—in all, numbering nearly four hundred males; he then dwelt in Chaldea. In absence of other as reliable evidence we must accept this testimony in regard to its origin, causes, and antiquity.

Voltaire, in his article on circumcision in his

Philosophical Dictionary, seems more intent on breaking down any testimony that might favor belief in any religion than to impart any useful light or information. He bases all his arguments on the book *Euterpe*, of Herodotus, wherein he relates that the Colchis appear to come from Egypt, as they remembered the ancient Egyptians and their customs more than the Egyptians remembered either the Colchis or their customs; the Colchis claimed to be an Egyptian colony settled there by Sesostris and resembled the Egyptians.

Voltaire claims that, as the Jews were then in a small nook of Arabia Petrea, it is hardly likely that, they being then an insignificant people, the Egyptians would have borrowed any of their customs. To read Voltaire's "Herodotus" is somewhat convincing, but Voltaire's "Herodotus" and Herodotus writing himself are two different things, and the book *Euterpe* says quite another thing from what M. Voltaire makes it say.

A perusal of Voltaire and a study of his Jewish critics on this subject, as found in the *Jews' Letters to Voltaire*, will convince any reader that as to circumcision M. Voltaire is an unreliable authority.

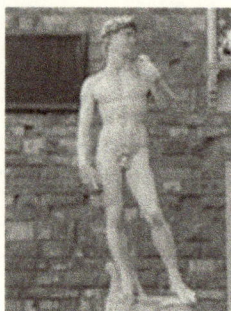

CHAPTER III—SPREAD OF CIRCUMCISION

From Chaldea, then, in the mountains of Armenia and Kurdistan, the practice of circumcision was, in all probability, first adopted by the Phoenicians, who finally relinquished the Israelitish rite as to age of performance and exchanged it for the Egyptian rite.

From Phoenicia its spread through the maritime enterprises of this race to foreign parts was easy. Egypt was the next place to adopt its practice; at first the priesthood and nobility, which included royalty, were the only ones who availed themselves of the practice.

The Egyptians connected circumcision with hygiene and cleanliness; this was the view of Herodotus, who looked upon the rite as a strictly hygienic measure. History relates of the existence of circumcision among the Egyptians as far back as the reign of Psammétich, who ruled toward the end of the sixth century B.C. The practice must then have been of a very religious and national nature, as we are told that Psammétich, having admitted some noted strangers, whom he allowed to dwell in Egypt without

54

being circumcised, brought himself into great disfavor among his subjects, and especially by the army, who looked upon an uncircumcised stranger as one undeserving of favors.

During the next century Pythagoras visited Egypt, and was compelled to submit to be circumcised before being admitted to the privilege of studying in the Egyptian temples. In the following century these restrictions were removed, for neither Herodotus nor Diodorus, who visited the country, were obliged to be circumcised, either to dwell among the people or to follow their studies.

There is one curious habit that is mentioned in connection with the rite of circumcision among these people, this being its relation to the taking of an oath or a solemn obligation. Among the Egyptians the circumcised phallus, as well as the rite of circumcision, seemed to be the symbol of the religious as well as of the political community, and the circumcised member was emblematical of civil patriotism as well as of the orthodox religion of the nation.

To the Egyptian, his circumcised phallus was the symbol of national and religious honor; and as the Anglo-Saxon holds aloft his right hand, with his left resting on the holy Bible, while taking an oath, so the ancient Egyptian raised his circumcised phallus in token of sincerity—a practice not altogether forgotten by his descendants of to-day. It was partly this custom of swearing, or of affirming, with the hand under the thigh, by the early Israelites, that caused many to believe that their circumcision was borrowed from the Egyptians, especially by M. Voltaire, who insists that it was the phallus that the hand was placed on, and that the translation has not the proper meaning, as given in the Bible.

Among the Arabs it was the practice to circumcise at the age of thirteen years, this being the age of Ishmael at his circumcision by his father, Abraham. The Arabs practiced circumcision long before the advent of Mohammed, who was himself circumcised. Pococke mentions a tradition which ascribes to the prophet the words,

> *Circumcision is an ordinance for men, and honorable in women.*

Although the rite is not a religious imposition, it has spread wherever the crescent has carried the Mohammedan faith. Uncircumcision and impurity are to a Mohammedan synonymous terms. Like the Abyssinians, the Arabs also practice female circumcision—an operation not without considerable medical import, as will be explained in the medical part of the work. This practice is also common in Ethopia.

Some authorities argue, from this association of female circumcision among the Southern Arabs, Ethiopians, and Abyssinians, that they did not derive their rite from the Israelites; but there is not much room for doubt but that the operation came down to the Arabians from Abraham through his son Ishmael. Considering the occupancy of Syria, Arabia, and Egypt by the French, and the intercourse with these countries by the British, it is surprising that the profession in the early part of the present century had not full information regarding the nature and objects of female circumcision as practiced in these countries. Delpesh observes, in relation to the Oriental practice, that his information was too vague to determine whether it was the nymphæ or the clitoris that were removed, or whether it was only practiced in cases of abnormal elongations of these parts.

M. Murat, however, writes at length on the subject, very intelligently, as well as Lonyer-Villermay, who, writing in the same work with Delpesh, thinks it is certainly the clitoris that is removed.[12] In Arabia, the trade or profession of a *resectricis nympharum* or she-circumciser is as stable an occupation with some matrons as that of cock-castration or caponizing is the sole occupation of many a matron in the south of Europe. It is related by Abulfeda that, in the battle of Ohod, where Mohammedanism came very near to a sudden end by the crushing defeat of the prophet and his followers, Hamza, the uncle of the prophet, seeing in the opposing ranks a Koreish chief, whom he knew, thus called out:

Come on, you son of a she-circumciser!

As Hamza was among the slain, it is most likely that he met his death from the hands of the chief, whose mother really followed that occupation. So extensive is the practice, that these old women sometimes go through a village crying out their occupation, like itinerant tinkers or scissors-grinders.

---

[12] *Dictionaire des Sciences Médicales*. Par une Société de médecins et de Chirurgiens. Paris, 1826, 60-volume edition.

The present ceremonies attending the performance of the rite among the Arabians are well described by Dr. Delange, a surgeon of the French army, as witnessed by him in the province of Constantine, in Algeria.

With these Arabs, circumcision is performed on a whole class, so to speak, at the same time, regardless of the trifling differences in their ages. It is preceded by feasting, the total length of the feast being for eight days. For the first seven days, all the Arabs of the quarter where the candidates for circumcision reside dress in their best. The poor have their mantles and clothes carefully washed, and the rich deck themselves out in their gold and silver brocaded vests and pantaloons.

During these seven days there is general rejoicing, and the Arabs spend most of this time in the village street, racing, firing guns, or engaging in sham battles between the different camps, during which one carries the green, or sacred banner, which is supposed to render the bearer invulnerable. The battle ends by the standard-bearer being fired at by all parties, and falling, but quickly rising again and waving the flag in token of its protecting power.

The Arabs now adjourn to another public place, where the notables and strangers are furnished seats on carpets; here a dance to the music of tumtums and the singing of invisible females takes place, the dancers being only males.[13]

---

[13] Dr. Delange mentions a peculiar social habit or custom among a tribe of Arabians that in a sociological sense is worth mentioning. He observes that for these dances

In the evening the women sing, to which the men listen in silence, this concert being kept up until midnight. On the seventh day, the women, decked out in their best, and with all their personal ornaments, accompanied by all the young men, armed with their guns and pistols, repair to the extremity of the oasis, where they gather plates of fine sand. With this sand they return to the village, where it is exposed overnight

---

females are preferred, but owing to the peculiar habit about to be related it is impossible to have any of the village women in Algeria assist at this part of the festivities; hence the men have to do the dancing. It appears that the females of one tribe—this being the tribe of Ouleds-Nails, who live on the southern borders of Algiers—are in the habit, when young, of emigrating to the oases of the Sahara, which are occupied by the French and traveling Arabs, where they give themselves up to a life of prostitution. After having exercised this life for some years they return to the tribe with a dowry in money, besides an ample supply of clothes and jewelry—the result of their economy—which enables them to contract favorable marriages. This practice is so common in this one particular tribe, and so much have they monopolized the profession of courtesan, that the name of the tribe of Ouleds-Nails is in Arabia synonymous with that of courtesan. These young women dance every evening in the Arab cafés, and are at times employed to do the dancing at Arab feasts. For this reason no self-respecting Arab woman ever allows herself to dance in public, or why the practice of both sexes dancing together is not practiced in Algerian villages, as a man would thereby consider himself disgraced.

—Dr. Delange, in *Receuil de Mémoires de Médecine de Chirurgie et de Pharmacie Militaire*, No. 105, August, 1868.

to the glare of the full moon on the terraces of the house. This last day closes with a grand banquet, given by the rich whose children are about to be circumcised, to which all the people are invited.

The next morning all the relatives of the candidates repair to the house where the rite is to be performed; the women going up into the second floor, wherefrom they can look down into the court from a porch screened with lattice-work, without themselves being seen. The men gather together on the ground-floor, together with the operator and his assistants and the children about to be circumcised, who are dressed in yellow, silken gowns. The child to be operated upon is seated in a pan of sand, while an assistant fixes his arms and holds the thighs well separated from behind.

The circumciser then examines the prepuce, the glans, and removes any sebaceous collection. This done, a compress with an aperture to admit of the passage of the glans is slipped over the organ; a small piece of leather, some six centimetres in diameter, with a small hole in the centre, is now used, the free end of the prepuce being drawn through the aperture; a ligature of woolen cord is then tied on to the prepuce next to the front of the leather shield, and, the knife being applied between the thread and the leather, the prepuce is removed at one sweep; the mucous inner layer is then lacerated with the thumb-nails and turned back over to join the other parts.

The surface is then sprinkled with *arar* or *genevriere* powder and dressed with a small cloth bandage, the subsequent dressings consisting of *ara* powder and oil. During the operation the women in the gallery keep up an unearthly music by means of tumtums, cymbals, and all the kettles and saucepans of the neighborhood, which are brought into requisition for the occasion. This music is accompanied with songs and chants, each woman striking out with an independent song of her own, either improvised or suggested by the occasion. This not only serves to drown the cries of the children, but it must, in a manner, assist to draw them away from the immediate contemplation of their sufferings. The prepuces are now gathered together and carried to the end of the oasis, where they are buried with ceremony and rejoicings. This circumcision only takes place once in three or four years, and the children are from four to eight years of age; of fifteen circumcised at the feast witnessed by M. Delange, only two had passed their eighth year.

In a very interesting old book, [14] *The Treaties of Alberti Bobovii*, who was attached to the court of Mohammed IV, published with annotations by Thomas Hyde, of Oxford, in 1690, there is a description of the Turkish performance of the rite which leads one to infer that they circumcised the children quite young:

Et cum puer præ dolore exclamat, imus ex duobus parentibus digitis in melle ad hoc comparato os ei obstruit; cæteris spectatoribus acclamantibus. O Deus, O

---

[14] *Tractatus, Alberti Bobovii, Turcarum Imp. Mohammedis IV olim Interpretis primarii, De Turcarum Liturgia, peregrinatione Meccana, Circumcisione, Ægrotorum Visitatione, etc. Oxonii, 1690.*

Deus, O Deus. Interim quoque Musica perstrepit, tympana et alia crepitacula concutiuntur, ne pueri planctus et ploratus audiatur.

Bobovii says that the age at which circumcision is performed is immaterial provided the candidate is old enough to make a profession of faith—which, however, is made for him by the godfather—in the following words:

There is no God but God, and Mohammed is his Prophet

or, as rendered by our author,

Non esse Deum nisi ipsum Deum, et Mohammedem esse Legatum Dei.

To which he adds that the child must not be an infant, but that he must be at least eight years of age. Like to the Arabs, the Turks celebrated the occasion by feasts, plays, and a general good time; the child was kept in bed for fifteen days to allow complete cicatrization to take place. The circumcision was performed with the boy standing.

Michel Le Feber, writing in 1681,[15] speaks of the tax levied on the Christians by the Turks, that they, the Christians, may enjoy liberty of conscience, and observes that, circumcision not being compulsory

---

[15] Michel Le Feber. *Le Theatre de la Turquie.* Paris, 1681.

among the Turks, it often led to trouble and annoyances, as many of the Turks evaded the operation.

The tax-gatherers in Turkey are very industrious, and, as being circumcised was, as a rule, sufficient evidence of not being a Christian, he often witnessed on the streets scenes wherein strangers, arrested by these tax-collectors, were compelled to show their circumcision as an indisputable sign of their exemption from the tax. He also relates that in their zeal for converts to Mohammedanism the Turks often resorted to presents to induce Christians to embrace their faith.

While in Aleppo, he saw a Portugese sailor, who, through presents, had forsaken his religion, but who had repented in the most emphatic manner when brought to face circumcision. Finding entreaties in vain, the Cadi ordered the immediate administration of a stupefying draught, and the sailor was then seized and circumcised without further ceremony.

In cases where the new Mohammedan is reasonable and submits like a hero, the ceremonies are more elaborate. Le Feber relates that if the candidate is a man of note or wealth he is mounted on a horse and exhibited all over the city; he is dressed in the richest of Turkish robes and in his hand he holds an arrow with the point directed to the sky; he is followed by a great concourse of people, some dressed in holiday attire and others in fantastic costumes; and general feasting and enjoyment is the rule over the course of the march, where all the people run to swell the crowd.

If the man happens to be a poor man, he is simply

hurriedly marched about on foot, with a simple arrow in his hand pointed skyward, to distinguish him from ordinary mortals; before him a crier proclaims in a loud voice that the new religionist has ennobled himself by professing the faith of the prophet in this solemn manner. A collection for his benefit is taken up among the booths and shops, which is mostly appropriated by the conductor, circumciser, and his assistants, after which he is circumcised without further ado.

The same author describes the operation as performed on the young Turks and the accompanying ceremonies. They differ in some respects from those employed in circumcising a convert. The parents of the child give a feast in proportion to their means, to which are invited the relatives of the family and personal friends; if of the upper ranks, he is promenaded about the town to the music of drums and cymbals, dressed in rich attire; two warriors lead the procession with drawn swords, and a troop of females who sing songs of joy bring up the rear; the procession now and then stops, when the two gladiators in the front indulge in a fierce set-to, hacking at each other in the most determined and murderous manner, but so studiedly shammy that neither is injured; on the return to the house, the child, who is usually eight or ten years of age, is bound hand and foot to prevent his causing any injury to himself, laid on a bed, and circumcised with a razor, the operation being performed either by a surgeon or the chief of a mosque.

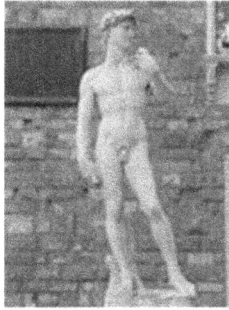

CHAPTER IV—CIRCUMCISION AMONG SAVAGE TRIBES

E. Casalis,[16] who, in the capacity of missionary, for a very long time resided among the Bassoutos, tells us that among that nation the operation is performed at the age of from thirteen to fifteen years. The ceremony is gone through once in three or four years.

So important an event is it considered by the Bassoutos that they date events from one of these observances, as the Romans dated events from a certain consulship, or the Greeks from an Olympiade. At the time fixed, all the candidates go through a sham rebellion and escape to the woods; the warriors arm and give chase, and, after a sham battle, capture the insurgents, whom they bring back as prisoners, amidst dancing and great rejoicings, which are the preludes to the feast.

---

[16] *La Circoncision, Sa Signification Social et Religieuse.* Par M. Paul Lafargue, in *the Bulletins de la Société d'Anthropologie de Paris.* Tome x, 3d fascicule, Juin à Octobre, 1887.

The next day the huts of mystery (*mapato*) are erected, where, after the circumcision, the young men are to reside for some eight months, under the tutorship of experienced teachers, who drill them in the use of the spear, sword, and shield, teaching them to endure hunger, thirst, blows, and all manner of hardships; prolonged fasts and cruel flagellations being regarded as pastimes between the exercises.

The severity of the regulations may be judged from the fact that the instructors have a right to put to death any one who may try to escape from these ordeals. The women are rigorously excluded from these camps, but the men are allowed to visit them, when they have the privilege of assisting the teachers by adding additional blows and precepts to the backs of the unlucky candidates.

After eight months of such training, the young men are oiled from head to foot and dressed in a garment, and are now given the name which they are to bear for the rest of their lives. The *mapato*, or mystery hut, is now burned to the ground and the young men return to the village.

The maternal uncle of the youth here presents him with a javelin for his defense, and a cow that is to furnish him with nourishment. Until the time of his marriage, the newly circumcised dwell together; their duties being of a menial character, such as gathering wood and attending to the flocks and droves.

M. Paul Lafargue looks upon circumcision among the negro races as being a rite commemorating their advent to manhood; Livingstone, who has also observed the above, related incidents in relation to the performance of *boguera*, or circumcision, among the

Bassoutos, believes that with them the rite has a purely civil significance, being in no way connected with religion.

Among many of the African tribes the young maids have an ordeal approaching to circumcision that they must pass when near the age of thirteen, this rite bearing precisely the same relation regarding their entrance into the state of womanhood that male circumcision denotes the entrance into manhood on the part of the males among the Bassoutos.

At the appointed time the maids are gathered together and conducted to the riverbank; they are placed under the care of expert matrons. They here reside, after having undergone a kind of baptism; they are maltreated, punished, and abused by the old women, with a view of making them hardy and insensible to pain; they are also schooled in the science and art of African household duties.

Among the Gallinas of Sierra Leone, in addition to the other observances, the clitoris of the young maid is excised at midnight, while the moon is at its full, after which they receive their name by which they are to be known through life. The initiation of each sex into these mysteries is exclusively for the sex engaged, and it would be as fatal for a man to steal into the camp of the women during the performance of these ceremonies as it would be fatal for a woman to enter a *mapato* where the young men are undergoing their ordeal. After their initiation into womanhood, the maids live by themselves, similarly to the young men, until they marry.

Lafargue relates that among the Australians circumcision is held in such importance that tribes at war will suspend all hostilities and meet in peace during the observance or performance of the rite. Here, again, we have a repetition, with a slight variation, of the practices of the Bassoutos—something which gives some countenance to the hero-warrior idea of the origin of circumcision advanced by Bergmann. The Australian warriors go through a mimic battle, and, after a series of combats, finally capture the boys aged about from thirteen to fourteen years, whom they bear away amidst the cries and lamentations of the mothers and other female relatives, who, in their excess of grief, mutilate themselves by cutting gashes into their thighs, so that they bleed profusely.

The boys are, in the meantime, carried to some out-of-the-way place, where an old man, perched on a tree or some rising ground, through the means of a musical instrument made of a deal-board and human hair, announced that the rite is in process of performance, so that neither women nor children might approach.

Tufts of moss are placed in the axilla and on the pubis, to represent puberty, and among some tribes the skin of the penis is divided to the scrotum with a stone knife, while others content themselves with simply making a circular incision, which removes the prepuce, after the Jewish manner, the excised portion being placed as a ring on the median finger of the left hand.

The circumcised then takes himself to the hills or woods, and there remains until healed, carefully guarding himself against the approach of any female. After this the third part of the ceremonies takes place: the godfather of the youth opens a vein in his own arm, the circumcised youth is placed on all-fours, and an incision is made from the neck down as far as the lumbar region, and the blood of the godfather is made to flow and mingle with that of the godchild; this being in reality a bloody baptism, and a near relation to the blood-compacts of the Arabs.

The Malays, as well as the men of Borneo, are circumcised. The Battos likewise perform the rite. Among the Islanders they sometimes ligate the prepuce so that it drops off. Among the Battos the same object is reached by small bamboo sticks, between which the prepuce is fastened.

In New Caledonia and Tidshi the boys are circumcised in their seventh year. The Tonga Islanders split the prepuce on the dorsum with a piece of bamboo or of shell. In the Marquesas and Sandwich Islands the operation is superintended by the priests.[17]

---

[17] *Circumcision.* By A. B. Arnold. *New York Med. Record*, Feb. 13, 1886.

Peter Charles Remondino

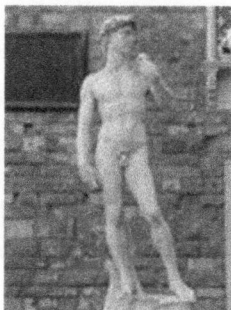

CHAPTER V—INFIBULATION, MUZZLING, AND OTHER CURIOUS PRACTICES

It seems a matter of controversy as to whether the Mexicans did or did not circumcise their children. That they had a blood-covenant is admitted by the historians, as well as the fact that this blood was taken from the prepuce; but that the prepuce was actually removed is something that is not agreed upon by all authorities.

Las Casas and Mendieta state that it was practiced by the Aztecs and Totonacs, while Brasseur de Bourbourg found traces of its practice among the Mijes. Las Casas states that on the twenty-eighth or the twenty-ninth day the child was presented to the temple, when the high-priest and his assistants placed it upon a stone and cut off the prepuce, the excised part being afterward burnt in the ashes.

Girls of the same age were deflowered by the finger of the high-priest, who ordered the operation to be repeated at the sixth year; and once a year, at the fifth month, all the children born during the year were scarified on the breast, stomach, or arms, to denote their reception as servants of their god.

Clavigero, on the other hand, denies that circumcision was ever practiced. It was customary in Mexico, according to most authorities, to take the children while infants to the temple, where the priests made an incision in the ear of the females, and an incision in the ear and prepuce of the males.[18]

Grotins and Arias Montan at one time advanced the idea that the western coast of South America was peopled by some mutinous sailors from the fleets of King Solomon, who, in their endeavor to go away far enough to be out of reach, were driven by winds and chance to the Peruvian coast.

Others have imagined that some of the lost tribes of Israel found their way eastward to America, by the way of China, to the Mexican coast. The same ideal tradition has made the lost tribes the fathers of the Iroquois Nation in the northeastern parts of the United States. An author, who will be quoted in another part of this work, scouts the idea that the rite, as performed in America, had any connection or common origin with the rite performed in Asia and Africa; but, true to his theory of the climatic causes of the origin of circumcision, he maintains that it originated here as it did elsewhere, being a performance born of climatic necessity.

He is, however, dissatisfied with Father Acosta for not being more explicit in relation to the *modus operandi* of the Mexican circumcision. The want of being explicit, and its consequences in this particular

---

[18] Bancroft's *Native Races*, vol. ii, page 278.

regard, may be inferred from a *Diatribe on Circumcision,* by a Mr. Mallet, in an encyclopædic dictionary of the last century, in which Mr. Mallet informs his readers that Mexicans were in the habit *of cutting off the ears and prepuces* of the newly born.

Herrera and Acosta agree with Clavigero in asserting that the Mexicans simply *bled* the prepuce. Pierre d'Angleria and other contemporary writers are as emphatic in asserting that in the island of Cosumel, in Yucatan, on the sea-board of the Gulf of Mexico and on the Florida coast, they have observed circumcision by the complete removal of the prepuce with a stone knife.

The Spanish monk, Gumilla, relates that the Saliva Indians of the Orinoco circumcised their infants on the eighth day. These Indians also included the females in the observance of the rite. The same author tells us of the barbarous and bloody performances, in relation to the rite, of the nations on the banks of the Quilato and the Uru, as well as those dwelling along the streams that empty into the Apure.

The same is said of the Guamo and of the Othomacos Indians; according to Gumilla, many of these Indians, in addition to the rite of circumcision, inflicted a number of cuts on the arms, legs, and over the body, to a degree that amounted to butchery, the child being reserved for this inhuman treatment until the age of ten or twelve years, that he might, by his greater powers of resistance and of recuperation, stand some chance of escaping alive from the ordeal.

The friar mentions that in 1721 he found a child dying from this treatment, the wounds having become gangrenous and the child dying of pyæmia; prior to the operation the children were stupefied with some narcotic drink, and were insensible during its performance.[19]

Besides circumcision, the Americans practiced several other operations that bore an analogy to the operation of infibulation, a procedure common to the Orient and to early Europe, and so ancient that, like circumcision, its source is in the misty clouds of antiquity. It consisted in introducing a large ring, either of gold, silver, or iron, through an opening made into the prepuce, the free ends being then welded together. Females were treated likewise, the ring including both labia. In some countries an agglutination of the parts induced by some irritant or a cutting instrument answered the purpose among females.

Dunglison mentions that the prepuce was first drawn over the glans, and then that the ring transfixed the prepuce in that position; that the ancients so muzzled the gladiators to prevent them from being enervated by venereal indulgence.

The ancient Germans lived a life of chastity until their marriage, and to their observance of a chaste life can be attributed the superior physical development of the race, as both males and females were not only fully developed, but were not enervated by either sexual excess or inclinations before having offspring, which were necessarily robust and healthy.

---

[19] *Recherches Philosophiques sur les Americains, ou Memoires Interessants pour servir à l'Histoire de l'Espece Humaine.* Par M. de P. Edition par Dom Pernety. Tome ii. Article, *Circoncision*, Berlin, 1774.

To obtain the same results in a nation given to indolence and luxury, and lax in its morality, some physical restraint was required, and we therefore find the practice of infibulation coming from the warm countries to the East. The ancients not only infibulated their gladiators to restrain them from venery, but they also subjected their chanters and singers to the same ordeal, as it was found to improve the voice; comedians and public dancers were also restrained from ruining their talents by the means of infibulation.

In an old Amsterdam edition of Locke's *Essay on the Extent of the Human Understanding,* there is a quotation from the voyages of Baumgarten, wherein he states having seen in Egypt a devout dervish seated in a perfect state of nature among the sand-hillocks, who was regarded as a most holy and chaste man for the reason that he did not associate with his own kind, but only with the animals.

As this was by no means an uncommon case, it led the Greek monks, in Greece and Asia Minor, to resort to every expedient to protect their chastity; in some of the monasteries not only were the monks muzzled by the process of infibulation, but they even had rules that excluded all females, either human or animal, from within their convent—a habit that still prevails among many of the convents of the Orient to this day—that on Mount Athos especially, omitting the infibulation of the ancients.

Readers living in the climates of extreme ranges and of seasonal change cannot understand the physical temptations that beset mortals in certain climates, any more than they can imagine the faultless condition of the climate itself. The subject of climatic influences will be more fully discussed further on; but climate, as a factor of habits and usages in one part of the world, that are incomprehensible to those living in others, plays a part that is but little appreciated or understood; whether it be the question of diet, dress, or custom, climate exerts its influence in no uncertain manner.

As Sulpicius Severus remarked to the Greek monks, when they accused the Gaulish monks with voracity and gluttony,

> *That which you of Greece consider as superfluous, the climate of Gaul renders into a positive necessity.*

So of all physical needs and passions—they are subject to a similar law. Those who have read Canon Kingsley's small work on the *Hermits of Asia, Africa, and Europe* will appreciate the above remarks; and it may be incidentally mentioned that his description of the climate that is common to the hilly country bordering on the eastern half of the Mediterranean Sea gives as vivid and as graphic a description of the physical condition of the climate and of its effects as can well be written.

It occurs in the life of the hermit Hilarion, and the description given relates to his last home in the ruins of an old temple, situated on a cliff in the island of Cyprus, where the air is so invigorating that "man needs there hardly to eat, drink, or sleep, for the act of breathing will give life enough." The work gives the best insight also into origin and causes that led to monachism, as well as it tells the benefit that the condition conferred on humanity, showing a phase in the march of civilization that is but little understood.

But, to return to the subject of infibulation, which has, in a manner, necessitated this digression from the main topic. Thwing [20] informs us that in ancient Germany woman was considered the moral equal of man, and that woman might traverse the vast stretches of country unprotected and unharmed. Woman never held such a position in the Oriental countries; neither has man, under the sub-tropics, a like self-command as shown by those ancient Gauls.

So that, with the advent of Christianity and the moral revolution that followed, primitive methods, either inflicted on others or self-inflicted, were adopted to insure a chaste life. Infibulation was known, as already stated, for centuries, and in those rude times it seemed as the most natural and effective mode of accomplishing the object. It was not as barbarous an operation as emasculation on the male, as it only temporarily interfered with his functions.

In the Old World the practice is still performed in various manners. In Ethiopia, when a female child is born the vulva is stitched together, allowing only the necessary passage for the needs of nature. These parts adhere together, and the father is then possessed of a virgin which he can sell to the highest bidder, the union being severed with a sharp knife just before marriage.

In some parts of Africa and Asia, a ring, as before

[20] *The Family, a Historical and Social Study,* Charles Franklin Thwing. Boston, 1887.

stated, transfixed the labia, which, to be removed, required either a file or a chisel; this is worn only by virgins. Married women wear a sort of muzzle fastened around the body, locked by means of a key or a padlock, the key being only in the possession of the husband.

The wealthy have their seraglios and eunuchs, that take the place of the belt and lock. Another method is a mailed belt worn about the hips, made of brass wire, with a secret combination of fastenings, known only to the husband. In the museum in Naples are to be seen some of these belts, studded with sharp-pointed pikes over the abdominal part of the instrument, which was calculated to prevent even innocent familiarity, such as nest-hiding, to say nothing of greater evils.

In the *Les Femmes, Les Eunuchs, et Les Guerrieres du Soudan*, Col. Du Bisson mentions a very peculiar custom invented by the careful jealousy that is inseparable from harem life. He had noticed that many of the harem inmates, contrary to the general Oriental custom, were allowed to go about unattended by the usual guard of eunuchs, but that they walked in a painful, hesitating, and impeded manner.

This walk was not the conventional, short, shuffling step that peculiarity of dress and shoe-wear imposes on the Japanese beauty, nor the willowy, swaying gait produced in the Chinese beauty by the lack of a sufficiency of foot; neither could it be ascribed to the presence of the ancient jingling chain of bells which induced the mincing steps of the virgins of Judea—an invention which confined the lower limbs within certain limits by being worn just below the knees, and calculated to prevent the rupture of the hymen by any undue length of step or violent exercise; hence a tinkling noise and a mincing step always denoted a virgin.

In Du Bisson's cases, however, virgins were out of the question; they might be the victims of enforced continence, but a Soudanese harem contains no virgins. On inquiry he learned that the very peculiar and unmistakably painful gait was due to the fact that each woman carried a bamboo stick, about eight inches in length, three inches or more being inserted in the vagina so as to effectually fill the opening, the balance projecting beyond, between the thighs of the person; this bamboo stick, or guardian of female virtue, was held in place by a strap with a shield that covered the vulva, the whole apparatus being strapped about the hips and waist, and the whole being held in an undisplaceable position by a padlock.

This was affixed to the woman whenever she was allowed outside the harem grounds, being placed in position by the eunuch, who carried the key at his girdle. In such a harness virtue can be considered perfectly safe; even safe from any mental depredation or revolution, as, with the plug causing such uncomfortable sensations, it is perfectly safe to infer that the imagination could not be seduced by any Don Juanic or other Byronic unvirtuous revelry.

The physical ills that this contrivance must cause are necessarily without number, as the instrument is not as lightly constructed as our modern stem pessaries; but to the Oriental who can replace a woman at any time and who prizes the virginity, continence, and chastity of his slaves, even if enforced, more than their health or their lives, these are matters of secondary importance. In the Soudan there are no divorce courts, hence the probable necessity of the apparatus, and, as the woman is not obliged to wear it unless she chooses to go out unattended, it can hardly be considered as a compulsory barbarity. In the United States such a practice might do away with considerable divorce proceedings.

Celsus gives a detailed description of the manner of infibulating as practiced among the Romans. According to this authority, it was employed by them on the youth attending the public schools, as well as upon the actors, dancers, and choristers, who were sold to the directors of the plays and spectacles. In the cabinet of the Roman College there are to be seen two small statues representing two infibulated musicians, which are remarkable for the excessive size of the ring and the leanness of the persons to which they are attached. The mode of applying this ring did not differ much from the usual method of preparing the ear for pendants.[21]

Among the Greek monks mentioned, the infibulation serves a manifold purpose; it not only is a sure badge of chastity, but its weight and size is very often increased so as to render it an instrument of penitence, and considerable rivalry exists at times in this regard.

Virey notices that the Hindoo bonze, or fakir, at times submits to infibulation at the same time that he

---

[21] *The Recherches Philosophiques sur les Americains* and Virey, in the 24th volume of the *Dictionaire des Sciences Médicales*, are very full on this subject, and for fuller information the reader is referred to those works.

takes his vows of eternal chastity. This ring is at times enormous, being sometimes six inches in diameter; so that it is a burden. These saints are held in great esteem and veneration.

Nelaton, in the sixth volume of his *Surgery*, mentions the case of a man who presented himself at Dupuytren's clinic with a tumefied, thickened, and somewhat dilapidated and ulcerated prepuce; this prepuce had worn a couple of golden padlocks for five years, a woman having thus infibulated his organ.

In an elaborate work on the subject of circumcision, [22] de Vanier du Havre relates, on the authority of M. Martin Flaccourt, that with the Madécasses the children are circumcised on the eighth day after birth; and that in some portions of the country the mother swallows the removed portion of the prepuce, while in others the father loads the prepuce in some form of fire-arm, which is afterward fired in the air.

In the neighborhood of Djezan, in Arabia, as reported by M. Fulgence Fresnel in the *Revue de Deux Mondes* of 1838, courtship and matrimony are not so great social events as they are with our society beaux. The occasion is probably considered social enough by the rest of the invited guests, but it can hardly be called an agreeable episode in the life of the groom.

Those whose bashfulness prevents them from contracting marriage in civilized communities can have the consolation of knowing that in far-off Arabia,

---

[22] *Cause Morale de la Circoncision des Israelites, Institution Preventive de l'Onanisme des Enfants.* Par le Docteur Vanier, du Havre. Paris, 1847.

among the fierce followers of the conquerors of Spain and of the Eastern Empire, they have sympathizing fellow-sufferers whom the conventionalities of the country deter from rushing into matrimony.

In this region, circumcision is performed on the adult at the time of his candidacy for matrimonial bliss. A more inauspicious occasion could not possibly have been chosen, unless as in another Mohammedan tribe, who circumcise the bridegroom on the day after his marriage and sprinkle the blood that falls from the cut onto the veil of the bride. The bride is present, and the victim is handed over to what might be called the executioner of the holy office, who proceeds to circumcise the victim in what might be called its utmost degree of performance and barbarity.

This attention does not stop at the pendulous and loose prepuce. He devotes himself to the skin of the whole organ; beginning at the prepuce he gradually works backward, removing the whole skin of the penis—a flaying alive, and nothing more. Should the victim betray any sign of weakness, or allow as much as a sigh or groan to escape him, or even allow the muscles of the face to betray the fact that he is not immensely enjoying the occasion, the bride elect at once leaves him for good, saying that she does not wish a woman for a husband. A large proportion of the male population annually die from this operation. So that the Arabs of the Djezin can be likened to those spiders who lose their life while in the act of copulation—the female making a dinner from off the male—only the spider is said to die a happy death, while that of the Arab is one of misery.

Margrave and Martyr have recorded a very peculiar

practice common among some South American tribes: A kind of a tube is fastened onto the prepuce by means of threads of the *tacoynhaa*, the latter being the bark of a certain kind of a tree. Cabras brought one of the natives, so muzzled, to Lisbon, on the return from his first voyage. Some tribes were observed to wear an apparatus like the old-fashioned candle-extinguisher, the virile member having been forced into this receptacle, which was strapped about the loins.

The travelers Spix and Martius found the practice of circumcision of both sexes in the region of the upper Amazon River and among the Tuncas. Squires mentions a curious custom of the aborigines of Nicaragua. They wound the penis of their little sons and let some of the blood flow on an ear of corn, which is divided among the assembled guests and eaten by them with great ceremony.

On the fifth day after birth it is the custom among the Omaha Indians of North America to christen the infant, the child being stripped and spotted with a red pigment; considerable ceremony accompanies the act.[23]

Among the cannibals of Australia, Lumholtz [24] observed a practice that seems to have no analogue in the wide world, either as an operation or in regard to its purposes. About ninety-five per cent. of the children are subjected to the ordeal. This is no less

---

[23] *Annual Report of the Bureau of Ethnology.* By J. W. Powell. Washington, 1881, 1882.

[24] *Among Cannibals, or Four Years' Travels in Australia.* By Carl Lumholtz. Page 46. Charles Scribner & Son, 1889.

than the formation of an artificial hypospadias; this abnormality is formed through the penis into the urethra, near its junction with the scrotum; the wound is about an inch in length and is made with a flint knife which serves for no other purpose; the edges of the wound are burned with a hot stone, and the wound is subsequently kept open by the introduction of a small piece of wood, which, on healing, leaves a permanent opening.

These cannibals undoubtedly are inspired by some Malthusian spirit which impels them thus to functionally eunuchize themselves in one sense, as during copulation the seminal discharge flies out backward through this opening, being thereby a most effectual check on further procreation.

By some, this practice has been attributed to the unreliability of the seasons in regard to food-production; but Lumholtz observes that where the practice is most in vogue—among the tribes to the west of the Diamantina River and west and north of the Gulf of Carpentaria—the food-supply is not deficient, the region being full of rats, fish, and vegetables. All the tribes are not subject to the practice of the operation at the same time of life; in some, the hypospadias is not produced until in adult life and after the person has married and has become the father of one or two children, when he must submit to the requirements of the law; the operation seems to be invested with some civil or religious significance, as a palisade or stockade of trees is placed around the place where it is performed.

A native, aged about twenty years, informed Lumholtz that the operation was performed because the blacks did not like to hear the children cry about the camp, and, further, that they were not desirous of having many children; this native had not yet become a father and had not yet been subjected to the operation. The natives were observed to be fat and in good physical condition.

There is something mysterious in this operation. It can easily be conceived how circumcision might at times have been suggested by its spontaneous and natural performance without any assistance from man.

Cullerier reports one case of partial circumcision through the means of an accident happening to a painter. The man was at work on a ladder, with a small bucket of paint hooked into one of the rounds above him; through some means the bucket lost its hold and in falling struck the penis on its dorsum with such force that the prepuce was cut through on a parallel with the corona of the glans for fully two-thirds of its circumference, the glans slipping through the opening and gathering in a fleshy bunch underneath the frenum.

This man carried this abnormality for some years, when, desiring to marry and seeing that this appendage would be as much of an impediment as one of the huge rings worn by the Hindoo devotee, he applied to Cullevier for advice, who promptly removed it with the knife.[25] The writer has seen three cases,

---

[25] These interesting historical facts in relation to the holy prepuce were published in the *Journal l'Excommunier* in January of 1870, when the writer was in France. They were contributed by A. S. Morin, of Miron, a learned historiographer and antiquary. Europe has not recovered

during his practice, of spontaneous circumcision, all resulting from phymosis as a secondary affection to venereal disease.

The first case occurred when he first entered into practice; it was in a young, stout, and full-blooded man with a violent gonorrhoea. There was much swelling and tumefaction of the whole organ, which seemed to be very rebellious to all treatment. At one of his morning visits he was horrified to observe a transverse, livid mark at what seemed to be the middle of the organ; by noon this had gained ground to the right and left and there was no mistaking that it meant nothing less than mortification.

Never having seen a case, the natural uncomfortable conclusion was that, through some cause or other or the natural result of excessive congestion, the man was about to lose one-half of his organ; and Burnside at Fredericksburg was in no greater state of suspense and uncertainty with the fate of the Army of the Potomac on his hands than the writer must acknowledge he was with this man and his organ apparently liquefying under his treatment.

The surprise can be better imagined than described when, on the following morning, the glans made its appearance safe and sound out of its

---

from its love of the supernatural that it had so strongly in the middle ages. The blood of St. Gennaro still liquefies once a year, and many churches still claim to possess the identical winding sheet that served our Lord prior to his resurrection, as well as more than one church has the holy cloth that St. Veronica used on the way to Calvary, which has an impression of the face of the Saviour.

imprisonment, and at right angles with the organ there hung the prepuce, thick and as large and as long as the penis itself, inflammatory deposit and infiltration having brought it to that shape and consistence; the glans became completely uncovered; the parts gathered underneath, where, in the course of some weeks, they had shrunk to the size of a walnut, which was afterward removed by the knife.

In this case, as in the other two cases observed, the corona was very prominent and acted as an internal tourniquet by its upward pressure, the line of demarcation being on the dorsum in the three cases noted.

That such cases would suggest circumcision is not only probable but possible, as it would point out the manner of performing the operation; but, in the cases of the Australian savages, who performed an artificial hypospadias on themselves for a specific purpose, requiring a knowledge of the anatomical relation of the parts as well as of their physiological functions, it is hard to speculate how the operation was first suggested or how it came at first to be performed.

As a Malthusian agent it is certainly an operation of the highest merit, and it should be introduced, by all means, in the United States, where the wealth and luxury in which the people dwell is fast drifting them toward the same whirlpool that engulfed Rome, which was preceded by a dislike to have children.

Whenever the writer sees the poor anæmic, broken-down victim of many miscarriages, he cannot help but feel that, if the laws of the Damiantina River savages were enforced on their husbands, it would be a blessing to the poor women without materially injuring the husbands, who, in case of need of a re-establishment of the functions of procreation, might be fitted with a vulcanite plate for the occasion—something like our cleft-palate patients are supplied with a plate that enables them to articulate.

It was the custom among the Hottentots, when first discovered or known to the whites, to remove one of their testicles. This was supposed to enable them to run more swiftly and to be lighter-footed in the race. The real reason, afterward found, was a mixture of pure humanitarianism and Malthusianism boiled down to Hottentot ethics.

With them a monorchid was not supposed to beget twins; when twins are born in the family, the mother generally smothers the female, if one happens to be such; if not, then the feeblest of the two is sacrificed. In their migratory and nomadic life the mother finds it impossible to either carry or care for the two children.

The male Hottentot, rather than have any avoidable infanticide in his family, or that his wife should go through and suffer the annoyance and pangs of an unnecessary and unprofitable pregnancy, generously has one testicle removed; this is something that the ordinary civilized white man would not do, even if his legitimate wife and all his outside concubines were to have twins or triplets every nine months; so that, even as strange as it may appear, civilization must need go to the wild Bushmen in search of that grand old Quixotic chivalry that was in ancient times always ready to sacrifice itself for the welfare of woman.

The old Greek and Roman statues, representing the gods and athletes of ancient Greece and Rome, are a puzzle to many, owing to the diminutive and phimosed virile organ that the artists have attached to them. Galen represents that the disuse of the organ by the athletes was the cause of its undeveloped form, and that as the organ of these did not figure in the worship of Venus, or participate in the festivals of Bacchus, but was used solely and simply for micturating purposes, impotence was often the result, citing the case of a patient who came to consult him for an obstinate priapism resulting from venereal excess, who met, in his anteroom, an athlete who was being treated for the opposite condition, due to the too rigid continence to which he had been for years subjected.

Acton does not believe that continued continence has that effect, quoting Dr. Bergeret, who had long been physician to a number of religious societies, as saying that he had never seen serious troubles of the organs of generation in these communities, which denotes that if they indulged in proper fasting and prayer they were in the same condition of flaccid impotence as the athlete in Galen's anteroom. Louis VII, of France, tried fasting and prayer in connection with rigid continence, and, as a result, his wife, Queen Eleonore, was divorced from him and married Henry II, of England, who had not been continent.

Hence, we see that the old sculptors, whether wishing to represent Jupiter or Plato, Æsculapius or Mars, a strongly knit and muscular frame was desired, an athlete, gladiator, or soldier being used as a model; the small, puerile, funnel-prepuced organ belonged to all these muscular or well-trained classes, was a natural appendage, as enforced continence and the most absolute chastity was the rule, to enforce which they even resorted to infibulation.

This enforced continence often resulted in impotence, even before the prime of life was passed, accompanied by an inevitable atrophy of the male organ, with the resulting prepuce in the shape in which it is found in a boy of from eight to twelve years, precisely as they are found on the statues. How faithful the sculptors and artists were to nature and life in their representations can well be imagined by a critical examination of the Apollo Belvidere, where the difference of the scrotal position that exists between the right and left testicles is carried out to the minutest anatomical detail.

In our age it is hard to conceive why their most masculine men should be deified, and all their gods represented as the most perfect of bodily development, while at the same time the finest physical specimens of manhood were doomed to a life of the most rigorous continence. It is also astonishing that all this should be done not from any principle or consideration of morality or virtue, but simply as a means subservient in producing at its maximum the highest degree of physical development and endurance.

Peter Charles Remondino

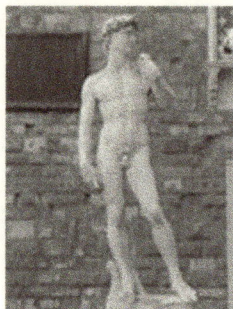

CHAPTER VI—ATTEMPTS TO ABOLISH CIRCUMCISION

Probably no rite or practice of a custom has been such a long-standing bone of contention as circumcision; nor does the Sphynx surpass this relic of bygone ages in mystery.

From time immemorial its practice has been the subject of disputes, and its literature finds oftentimes its friends and foes ranged side by side. At one time a noted Israelite and Voltaire, the scoffer of Judaism, may be consulted on the question as to whether Israelite or Egyptian is entitled to priority as to its original practice with a like answer; and, again, Christians are found who, after a careful investigation, will accord this to the Israelites.

In Rome, the persecuted Hebrew was stopped on the street and compelled to show the mark of circumcision, that he might be taxed, and in Turkish parts the Christian was subjected to the same indignity to enable the tax-gatherer to harvest the impost which he paid for his liberty of conscience and not being circumcised. When the monkish missionaries of the Catholic faith first entered Abyssinia, they were shocked to find their converts insisting on their time-honored practice of circumcision; and later, when the Propaganda sent its own missionaries, they were scandalized to see Christians practicing what they looked upon as an infidel rite; and nothing but the most earnest confession of faith, with the assurance that the rite of circumcision was only a physical remedy, and that in their conscience it in no wise possessed any religious significance, and that neither did they, in any sense, hold it in any connection with the sacrament of baptism, permitted these Abyssinians to save themselves from excommunication.

Later still, when an Abyssinian bishop was present in Lisbon, the clergy of the city refused him the right of celebrating the sacrifice of the holy mass in the Cathedral of Lisbon, on the ground that he, having been circumcised, was no better than a heretic. The Abyssinian Christians still practice the rite at the present day.

The Turks, although very fanatical and greater proselyters than the Christians of Rome, seem now and then to relax in favor of general utility, as we find Bajazet II writing to the Pope, Alexander VI, supplicating his Holiness to confer a cardinal's hat on the Archbishop of Arles as a special favor to the Turkish emperor, as he knew that the archbishop *had a secret leaning toward Mohammedanism.*

As the clergy of those days, from the Holy Father down, were more politicians than followers of the humble Nazarene, the heaven of Mohammed had probably more attractions for their taste than the ideal Christian paradise, and it is possible that the good archbishop would have submitted to a cardinal's hat and circumcision at the same time to secure the good things of this world and of those in the world to come.

History also relates that his most Christian majesty, Henry III, of France, as a relaxation to the interminable squabble between two Christian religious factions which were rending France, and which in the end cost him his life, actually wrote a letter to the Sultan, asking the favor to be allowed to stand as godfather at the circumcision of his son.

When it is remembered that the godfather at a Turkish circumcision has to make a strong profession of Moslem faith and the answers as sponsor for the child, and must promise that the child will be faithful to the Koran and Mohammed, it will be seen that, however much the lower levels of humanity may quarrel over trifles, the heads of the people easily accommodated themselves to any existing circumstances. Friar Clemens might as well have let such a liberal-minded monarch live, as any of the existing churches could easily have got along with him.

On the other hand, we have the remarkable tenacity to custom and habit in this regard, as exhibited by the Moslems, who, although having neither ordinance nor authority for its performance, either in their law, creed, or in any order from their prophet, still no more zealous circumciser exists than the son of Islam, who exacts from all proselytes the excision of the prepuce.

Mohammed was circumcised in his boyhood, and, although he did not order its performance to his followers, he did not see fit to proscribe a custom so general to the Arabians, where the greater development of the prepuce probably renders circumcision a necessity.

From the same reason it is easy to perceive why the rite has found such general observance among the Africans, who are as noted for long and leathery prepuces as for their slim shanks. One author, writing in 1772, in a work entitled *Philosophical Researches on the Americans*, treats the subject in a very intelligent manner. His arguments are both ingenious and plausible. This author looks upon circumcision as of purely climatic origin in its inceptive causes. From a careful survey of the natural history of man in his general distribution over the globe, he finds that circumcision may be said to be restricted to within certain boundaries of latitude, equidistant on both sides of the line.

No circumcised people have ever inhabited northern regions, and the bulk of the circumcised races are found within certain climates. From this reasoning it is easy to see why the rite should lose its standing under certain climatic conditions, unless bolstered up by some religious significance, as it is equally easy to foresee why it should flourish elsewhere, even without any religious backing or ordinance. It is well known that in Ethiopia and the neighboring countries, excrescences and elongation of either the prepuce or nymphæ are as probable as the existence of an enlarged thyroid gland or goitre among the inhabitants of some of the valleys of Switzerland or of those of the Tyrol.

According to the author of the treatise just quoted,

circumcision would be nothing more than a remedy to repair the evils that a faulty construction of the human body developed in certain climatic conditions.

With the Israelites it is observed as a religious rite, although they are not strangers to the physical benefits that circumcision confers upon them; the fact that even where no prepuce exists, as sometimes happens, the circumciser nevertheless goes on with the rite, being satisfied with drawing a few drops of blood from the skin near the glans, stamps the operation essentially as being a religious rite.

Persecutions have signally failed to suppress its performance by those of the Hebrew faith. Beginning with the decree of Antiochus, 167 B.C., which consigned every Hebrew mother to death who dared to circumcise her offspring, they have not ceased to suffer in defense of their rite.

Adrian, among other repressive measures, forbade circumcision; under Antonine this edict was still enforced, but he afterward recalled it and gave to the Hebrews the right of observing their religious rites. Marcus Aurelius, however, revived the edict of Adrian. Heliogabalus, who ascended the Roman throne in the year 218 A.D., was himself circumcised.

During the reign of Constantine all the laws that interfered with Hebraic rites were renewed, with the addition that any Hebrew who should circumcise a slave should suffer death. Under the sway of Justinian, in the sixth century, the persecutions against these people were so oppressive that a Hebrew was not allowed to raise or educate his own child in the faith of his fathers. In the seventh century, the augurs having prophesied the ruin of the Roman Empire by a circumcised race to the emperor Heraclius, the persecutions were renewed against these unfortunate people.

In this century, Hebrews refusing baptism suffered banishment and confiscation of all their property; they were obliged to renounce the Sabbath, circumcision, and all Hebraic rites if they wished to remain.

About this period the success of the Saracens induced persecutions of the Hebrews in Spain, where their children were taken away from them that they might be raised in the Christian religion. In the fifteenth century they suffered the greatest persecution and martyrdom at the hands of the Spanish Inquisition.

The persecutions above cited were national and governmental persecutions leveled directly at the Jewish nation and creed; the persecutions that they momentarily suffered at other times had no signification beyond the exhibition of popular spite and fury, but those above cited were moves calculated to extirpate the creed, if not the people, from off the face of the globe. If repressive measures are of any avail, circumcision as an Hebraic rite should now have no existence. Its present existence and observance show a vitality that is simply phenomenal; its resistance and apparent indestructibility would seem to stamp it as of divine origin.

No custom, habit, or rite has survived so many ages and so many persecutions; other customs have died a natural death with time or want of persecution, but circumcision, either in peace or in war, has held its own, from the misty epochs of the stone age to the present.

Peter Charles Remondino

There is something pathetic and soul-appealing in contemplating the early Christians forced to worship in the catacombs of Rome, hunted like wild animals in their subterranean burrows, and then given the choice of making offerings to the heathen gods or being thrown into the arena as prey to wild beasts; so are we stirred when we think of the Spanish Jew, who had made Spain his home for centuries, being driven into exile in such droves that no country could receive them; we see them perishing of hunger by the thousands on the African coast, and dying of starvation on the quays of the ports of civilized Italy.

That many, through all these trials, were forced to embrace other religions is not astonishing. In Spain apostacy was to no purpose, as the Inquisition could not be expected to split hairs in regard to an apostate Jew, when it sent the best of Gothic blood, raised in the Catholic faith, to the *auto da fé* or the scaffold—the rack respecting neither faith nor profession that fell into its clutches. In milder persecutions, however, he escaped by outwardly conforming to the demands of his oppressors and history tells us of the circumcisions secretly performed on the dead Jew, that the spirit of the law of their fathers might be carried out.

In other cases, threatened exile, confiscation, or exorbitant taxation drove them to adopt every possible expedient to eradicate the sign of their Israelitism and make attempts to reform a prepuce.

The first attempts in this line were made during the reign of Antiochus, when a number of Hebrews wished to become as the people about them who were not persecuted—*fecerunt cibi præputia.* This is no easy operation, and in later times by the aid of appliances, both in Rome and in Spain, they undertook to cause the skin to recover the glans. Martial, in speaking of the instrument used in Rome, a sort of a long funnel-shaped copper tube in which the Hebrew carried his virile organ, terms it *Judæm Pondum*, the weight of which, by drawing down the skin, was supposed in time to draw it down far enough to answer the purpose.

The apostle Paul, in his epistle to the Corinthians, refers to these practices when he says,

> *Was any one called being circumcised, let him not be uncircumcised.*

The operation of reforming a prepuce, or of obliterating the marks of circumcision, does not appear to have been a success.

The writer had one experience that was interesting. On one occasion he advised circumcision for the relief of a reflex nervous disease, in a tall, athletic Austrian sailor from the Adriatic; although the nature of the operation was explained to the man, he evidently did not appreciate its full nature and importance until a sweeping cut with a scalpel left the excised prepuce in the operator's hand. Most Adriatic sailors have sailed up the Bosphorus and are more or less familiar with both the Greek and Turkish nations; the latter they despise with gusto, *porchi di Turci* being the affectionate appellation they bestow on their national neighbors.

No sooner did he perceive the real condition of affairs than he began to beat his head, saying that he was disgraced forever, as he never would dare to associate with his countrymen again, as he would be liable to be taken for a *porcho di Turco*; his frenzy increased to such a pitch that to spare any unpleasantness it was deemed advisable to replace the prepuce, which was done accordingly, the man making a tolerable good recovery, as far as the grafted prepuce was concerned.

It required a secondary operation to overcome some cicatricial contraction, and, on the whole, he had a very serviceable prepuce; but, what was more to the point, it prevented his ever being mistaken for a Turk.

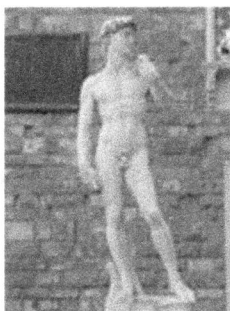

CHAPTER VII—MIRACLES AND THE HOLY PREPUCE

What strange fancies have circled themselves about the subject of generation or its organisms during the different stages of moral civilization since the world has existed! The efforts in this regard among different creeds have been something peculiar. Neither Mohammedans nor Hebrews—both zealous circumcisers—ever went to the lengths reached by Christian churches and their followers in some particulars concerning this rite; this being especially strange when it is considered that the new creed was the one that abolished the rite and through which the Jews suffered such cruel and unjust persecutions.

The early Christian Church celebrated and continues to celebrate the Feast of Circumcision, and history relates some strange events in connection with this circumcision. Having abolished and repudiated the rite, it would seem inconsistent that it should celebrate its performance on any occasion and consider such an event sufficiently memorable that its occurrence should excite the veneration of the church and be the means of exciting the pious zeal of the faithful. The strangest events in this connection are still more mysterious and incomprehensible, if not amusing, the only excuse for the occurrence being the greedy thirst for relics of any and all kinds that in the middle ages pervaded Europe.

At some remote period—in the thirteenth or fourteenth century—the abbey church of Coulombs, in the diocese of Chartres, in France, became possessed in some miraculous manner of the holy prepuce. This holy relic had the power of rendering all the sterile women in the neighborhood fruitful—a virtue, we are told, which filled the benevolent monks of the abbey with a pardonable amount of pride.

It had the additional virtue of inducing a subsequent easy delivery, which also added to the reputation and pardonable vanity of the good monks. This last virtue, however, we are told, came near causing the loss to the abbey of this inestimable prize, for, as a French writer observes, a too great reputation is at times an unlucky possession; at any rate, the royal spouse of good and valiant King Henry V—he of Agincourt, whom England waded up to its knees in the sea at Dover to meet on his return from that campaign—had followed the example of all good dames and was about to give England an heir.

Henry then governed a good part of France. Having heard of the wonderful efficacy of the relic of Coulombs, he early one morning threw the good monks into consternation by the arrival at the convent gate of a duly equipped herald and messenger from his kingship, asking for the loan of the relic with about as much ceremony as Mrs. Jones would ask for the loan of a flat-iron or saucepan from her neighbor, Mrs. Smith.

The queen, Catherine of France, was of their own country and Henry was too powerful to be put off or refused; there was no room for evasion, as the holy prepuce could not be duplicated; so the poor monks with the greatest reluctance parted with their precious relic, entrusting it into the hands of the royal envoy, which wended its way to London, where it in due time, being touched by the queen, insured a safe delivery.

Honest Henry then returned the relic to France; but so great was its reputation that royalty caused a special sanctuary to be erected for its reception, and a full period of twenty-five years occurred before the monks of Coulombs again regained possession of their prize, during which period the population of the neighborhood must have suffered from the natural increase of sterility and the physicians must have reaped a rich harvest owing to the increased difficulty and complications of labor induced by the absence of the relic.

On its return, the relic was found to have lost none of its virtues, and the good people and monks were all correspondingly made happy; in 1870, when the writer was in France, it was still working its miracles. Balzac found ample facts to found his famous "Droll Stories" without straining his imagination.

So great an attraction was not to go without attempted rivalry or imitators; hence we find in the *Dictionary of Moreri*, edition of 1715, in the third volume, at page 108, that several other establishments claim the honor of a like relic—namely, the Cathedral of Puy, in Velay; the collegial church of Antwerp; the

Abbey of our Saviour, of Charroux; and the Church of St. John Lateran, in Rome.

All of these have had very adventurous histories. The Abbey of Charroux was founded by Charlemagne in 788, and among the relics with which that monarch endowed the abbey the principal one was a fragment of the holy prepuce. This abbey enjoyed great reputation, and indulgences were granted by Papal bull to all those who assisted at the adoration of the relics. In the internecine wars of the sixteenth century the abbey fell into the hands of the godless and heretical Huguenots and the holy relic disappeared.

In 1856, while some workmen were at work demolishing an ancient wall on the abbey site, they discovered some relic cases. The bishop was at once notified, who immediately proceeded to investigate, when, lo and behold! there, sure enough, was a piece of desiccated flesh, with marks of coagulated blood; nothing more or less than the lost prepuce—long lost, but now found.

It was placed in charge of the Ursuline Sisterhood, where it has remained ever since undisturbed, except by a controversy in regard to the propriety of the relic, in which the good bishop ambled about in the most ambiguous manner, the only clearly defined portion of his dissertation being the one wherein he laments:

> ...the decadence of that truly Christian spirit which animated the laity of the middle ages with a radiant zeal. A piety also pervaded those gentle Christians of former times, who were possessed of a religious instruction which determined for

them the tenets of the creed and its practices—a happy state or condition of affairs, which prevented the intelligence of the faithful from wandering into the sloughs of unprofitable skepticism.

This settled the question as to the propriety of the prepuce being converted into a miracle-working relic; at least, as far as the good bishop was concerned.

It would be an injustice not to mention the other shrines in detail after the prominence that has been given to the abbeys of Coulombs and Charroux; so the history of another will be given. We are not told just how the Church of St. John Lateran in Rome first became possessed of *its* holy prepuce, but it nevertheless had one; also the only authentic one in existence, like all the others. It disappeared at one of the periodical sackings that Rome has repeatedly suffered at the hands of Goth, Vandal, or Christian. This time it was the soldiery of the eldest son of the church—Charles V—who did the sacking; it was in the year 1527, a soldier—probably some impious, heathenish mercenary—broke into the holy sanctuary of the church and stole therefrom the box that contained the holy relics, among them the holy prepuce.

These impious wretches, as a rule, came to grief in short order; hence we are told that this mercenary and sacrilegious soldier was compelled to secrete his box, when only a short distance from Rome, where the box remains and the mercenary wretch disappears, probably carried off bodily by the devil, as he deserved. Thirty years afterward the box is discovered by a priest, who, ignorant of its contents, carries it to the lady on whose domain it was found.

On being opened it was found to contain a piece of the anatomy of Saint Valentine, the lower jaw of Saint Martha, with one tooth still in place, and a small package upon which the name of the Saviour was inscribed. The lady picked up the package, when immediately the most fragrant odor pervaded the apartment, being exhaled by the miraculous packet, while the hand that held it was seen perceptibly to swell and stiffen; investigation proved it to be the holy prepuce stolen by the miscreant mercenary from St. John Lateran.

It is related that in 1559, a canon of the church of St. John Lateran, impelled by a worldly curiosity untempered by piety, undertook to make a critical examination of this relic, in the process of which, to better satisfy himself, he had the indiscretion to break off a small piece; instantly the most dreadful tempest broke over the place, followed by crashing peals of thunder and blinding flashes of lightning; then a sudden darkness covered the country, and the luckless priest and his assistants fell flat on their sacerdotal noses, feeling that their last hour had arrived.[26]

---

[26] This church has a remarkable history connected with its foundation. The tradition relates that in the dark ages some sacrilegious soldier had robbed a church in the neighborhood of its holy vessels of gold and silver. In the vessel in the Tabernacle there happened to be a consecrated wafer. The soldier journeyed on to Turin to dispose of his plunder, when, on arriving at the spot on which the church now stands, the wafer is said to have

Wonderful and miraculous cures are performed at these shrines, and some of the cures are of a nature that would baffle the intelligence of the most learned mind to ascertain the intricate and devious way that nature must at times journey to accomplish some of these changes. The writer well remembers seeing, in the Church of Corpus Christi, in Turin,[27] a long hall, covered, from marble pavement to ceiling, with votive tablets, after the manner inaugurated in the old temples of Greece. Modern votaries have the advantage of being able to record their cure, safe venture or escape from peril, by means of faithful representation of the event in painting or drawing, as the material and art is more common now than in the days of

---

ascended miraculously to some distance above the soldier's head, while at the same time the mule he rode, being imbued with more religious piety than his master, reverently knelt down on his front legs. The holy wafer was now encircled by a halo of shining light; this, with the kneeling donkey and the soldier raining blows on the pious animal, while he himself was unconscious of the presence of the host above him, attracted the attention of the populace, who apprehended the soldier, on whom the stolen vessels were found. The bishop in his pontificial robes, in solemn procession, received the consecrated wafer, which promptly descended into pious hands. The donkey was adopted by the bishop and the soldier was promptly hanged, in accordance with the general treatment of thieves in those days. The writer has more than once seen a flagstone inclosed within a railing that occupies the central spot of the floor or pavement of the church, it being the identical spot on which the donkey knelt.

[27] *Rush's Medical Inquiries*, vol. i, page 217.

ancient Greece, who recorded its cures by simple inscription in laconic terms.

Modern medicine labors under the disadvantage of presuming that the people are endowed with an intelligence that was unknown to ancient or mediæval people, when, in fact, the people are as credulous and as subject to imposition as they were in the earlier centuries of the present era.

With all its supposed superior intelligence, there is no fatter pasture for quacks and impostors than that presented by the people of the United States. Whenever I see the poor, intelligent, broad-minded physician struggling along, barely able to procure for himself the necessaries required to maintain himself with proper books and appliances, while the itinerant quack or dogmatic practitioner rolls in undeserved affluence, I question the wisdom of our ethical code.

Braddock, at the Monongahela, scorned to have his regulars, who had fought under Marlborough and Eugene, break ranks before a lot of breech-clouted savages, and take shelter that the nature of the ground and the trees could afford, thinking it an unfit action for men who had faced the veterans of Louis XIV on many a hard-fought European field. I sometimes think that if *our* regulars were, for only a season, to follow the example of the provincial militia at that battle, it would be better for the country, the people, science, and last, but not the least, for the profession.

The theory that we should not counsel with quacks is altogether mischievous and fallacious, although right and rigidly orthodox in its intent; were we to counsel and meet these gentry, we should expose their ignorance and assumption, and we should not be exposed to the charge of jealousy and of fear to meet them in consultation.

I remember on one occasion a client went to a lawyer for advice as to how he might dispossess some parties who had some adverse claim to some property which he owned, after due deliberation and a protracted siege of the house, in the vain hope of gaining admittance; the lawyer advised his client to go and nail up all exits and fasten them in, which had the effect of driving them out. So with our profession—we should not neglect an opportunity of meeting a quack in consultation, regardless of the nature of the case; it is the only way to nail them up; as it is, we have simply chained up the shepherd-dog and given the wolves full play.

The French Guards at Fontenoy, who out of courtesy refused to fire first on the English, may have been very ethical and chivalrous, but they were very foolish, as the English discharge nearly swept them from the field, and but for the Irish Brigade, who knew no ethics, Louis XV would in all likelihood have followed the example of King John, who, after Crecy, visited England for a season.

A disregard of ethics gave Copenhagen to Lord Nelson, who insisted on looking at Admiral Parker's signal to withdraw from action with his sightless eye, which could not see it.

A fear of disregarding ethics lost to Grouchy the chance of assisting Napoleon at Waterloo. In our strife against ignorance and quackery the profession should follow the general plan of action usually adopted by Lord Nelson—lie alongside of whom you can and sink or capture your enemy; let each man do his duty; never mind any general plan.

A reverse to this mode of fighting invariably lost the battle to the French and Spaniards, who were, as a rule, all tied up in ethical red tape. Our profession is broad, intelligent, and fearless; we do not profess any exclusive dogma, and should not, therefore, exclude persons; as a large ship throws its grappling-irons on to its adversary, we should always seek an opportunity to meet these gentry when practicable. As it is, we have placed them on the vantage-ground of appearing as being persecuted; our ethics need circumcising in this regard, and the prepuce of exclusion should be buried in the sands of the desert.

Moreover, we often are apt to learn something from even the most ignorant of these men. Rush investigated the nature of a cancer-cure by not refusing to meet and talk with one of this kind; [28] Fothergill learned from an old, unlicensed practitioner that there was a knowledge important to the physician beyond that picked up in the pathological laboratory or the study of microscopy; and that the practiced eye of an otherwise unlearned man could detect that there were general physical signs that negatived the unfavorable prognosis suggested by the presence of tube-casts. [29]

It is related of Sir Isaac Newton, that while riding homeward one day, the weather being clear and

---

[28] Fothergill. *Gout in its Protean Aspects*, page 158.

[29] *Philosophy of Magic*, from the French of Eusebe Salverte, vol. ii, page 143.

cloudless, in passing a herder he was warned to ride fast or the shower would wet him. Sir Isaac looked upon the man as demented, and rode on, not, however, without being caught in a drenching shower. Not being able to account for the source of information through which the rustic had gained his knowledge, he rode back, wet as he was, to learn something.

> My cow," answered the man, "always twists her tail in a certain way just before a rain, your Worship, and she so twisted it just before I saw you.[30]

Although twisting cow-tails do not figure in his "Principia," it is very probable that such a lesson was not without its remote effects on a mind like Newton's. A spider taught a lesson to one of Scotland's kings; so that one man may learn something from another.

Professor Letenneur, of the Medical School of Nantes, in his *Causerie à propos de la Circoncision,* mentions that the Convent of Saint Corneille, in Compiègne, claims to possess the identical instrument with which the Holy Circumcision was performed. Such a holy relic must have been unusually potential in performing many miracles.

In this connection it will not be amiss to notice the lapping over that the old phallic worship and idea has made on the new religions. It is also as interesting to observe how the human mind still leans toward observances and ideas which are believed to belong to

---

[30] *Dictionaire des Sciences Médicales.* Cullerier. Article, *Phimosis.* Vol. xli.

a solely pagan people. Hargrave Jennings, in a chapter devoted to phallic worship among the ancient Gauls, gives many interesting and curious examples, the first example that he notices being that of Saint Foutin (from whom the very expressive French word *foutre* is taken).

Foutin was the first Christian bishop of Lyons, and after his death, so intimately was priapic worship intermingled with the religion or theology of the Gauls, that somehow the memory of St. Foutin and the old, dethroned Priapus became commingled, and finally the former was unconsciously made to take the place of the latter. St. Foutin was immensely popular. He was believed to have a wonderful influence in restoring fertility to barren women and vigor and virility to impotent men. It is related that, in the church at Varages, in Provence, to such a degree of reputation had the shrine of this saint risen, it was customary for the afflicted to make a wax image of their impotent and flaccid organ, which was deposited on the shrine. On windy days the beadle and sexton were kept busy in picking up these imitations of decrepit and penitent male members from the floor, whither the wind wafted them, much to the annoyance and disturbance of the female portions of the congregation, whose devotions are said to have been sadly interfered with.

At a church in Embrun there was a large phallus, which was said to be a relic of St. Foutin. The worshippers were in the habit of offering wine to this deity—after the manner of the early Pagans—the wine being poured over the head of the organ and caught underneath in a sacred vessel. This was then called "holy vinegar," and was believed to be an efficacious remedy in cases of sterility, impotence, or want of virility.

Near the city of Bourges, at Bourg Dieu, there existed, during the Roman occupation of Gaul, an old priapic statue, which was worshipped by the surrounding country. The veneration in which it was held and the miracles with which it was accredited made it impolitic as well as impossible for the early missionaries and monks to remove it; it would have created too much opposition.

It was therefore allowed to remain, but gradually changed into a saint—St. Guerluchon—which, however, did not detract any from its former merit or reputation. Sterile women flocked to the shrine, and pilgrimages and a set number of days of devotion to this saint were in order. Scrapings from this statue infused in water were said to make a miraculous drink which insured conception.

Similar shrines to this same saint were erected at other places, and we are told that the good monks, who must have had an intense and lively interest in seeing that the population was increased, were kept busy supplying the statues with new members, as the women scraped away so industriously, either to prepare a drink for themselves or for their husbands, that a phallus did not last long.

At one of these shrines, so onerous became the industry of replacing a new phallus to the saint, that the good monks placed an apron over the organ, informing the good women that thereafter a simple contemplation of the sacred organ would be sufficient; and a special monk was detailed to take special charge of this apron, which was only to be lifted in special cases of sterility. By this innovation the good monks stole a march on their brothers in like shrines in other localities, such as those of St. Gilles, in Brittany, or St. Rene, in Anjou, where the old-fashioned scraping and replacing still was in vogue.

Near the seaport town of Brest, in Brittany, at the shrine of St. Guignole, the monks adopted a new expedient. They bored a hole through the statue, through which a phallus was made to project horizontally; as fast as the devotees scraped away in front the good monks as industriously pushed forward the wooden peg that formed the phallus, so that it gave the member the miraculous appearance of growing out as fast as scraped off, which greatly added to its reputation and efficacy.

The shrine continued in great vigor until the middle of the last century. Delaure mentions a similar shrine at Puy, also in France, which existed up to the outbreak of the French Revolution. The scrapings in this case were immersed in wine, and the guardians of the statue saw to it that no amount of paring or scraping should remove from the saint any of that appearance of vigor or virility which his great reputation demanded, this being done by a similar procedure as followed at the church near Brest, one of the attendants having been sent to investigate into the marvelous growth of the Brest phallus.

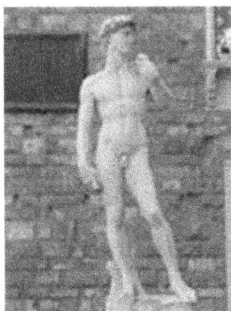

CHAPTER VIII—HISTORY OF EMASCULATION, CASTRATION, AND EUNUCHISM

For the earliest records in regard to emasculation we must go back to mythological relations.

In the old legendary lore of ancient Scandinavia or of Germany, the loves and hatreds of their semi-mythological heroes and heroines space over many romantic incidents before reaching a culmination. The swiftly flowing Rhine, with its precipitous banks, eddies, and rapids; the broad and more majestic Danube or Elb; the broad meadows and Druidical groves on its hilly slopes and stretches of dark and gloomy forest—all conspired to people the fancy with elfs, gnomes, fairies, and goblins, who were more or less intermingled in all the episodes that engaged their semi-mythological heroes.

This helped to fill in all their deeds with entertaining incidents; their halls and castles were made necessary accessories by the rigors of the climate, as well as were the beery feasts and carousals

113

with the inspiration of monotonous song also rendered necessaries by the same element; hence, we have various incidents, either entertaining or exciting, connected with their legendary tales, acting like periods of intermission between their love scenes, spites, hatreds, murders, and general cremations. From such material and such opportunities it was comparatively easy for Wagner to construct the thrilling and interesting incidents that compose his opera on the legend of the Nibelungenlied.

The Grecian landscape and topography does not permit of such richness of romantic incidents or details, any more than the love-making of the unfortunate spider who is devoured by his spidery Cleopatra at the end of his first sexual embrace could furnish any incidents for one of Amelie Rives's spirited novels; so that neither minstrel nor bard have recorded the details of the first emasculating tragedy, which from all accounts was a kind of an Olympian Donnybrook-fair sort of a paricidal-ending tragedy.

Unfortunately, Homer was not there to describe the event, or we might have had a Wagnerian opera with its Plutonic music to illustrate all its incidents; or even a Virgil could have made it into interesting verses; but, as it is, we must content ourselves with the laconic recitals that have been handed down by tradition, and, as all the Greek performances of those days were marked by an intense decisiveness, with an utter lack of circumlocution, it is probable that there was not much to relate beyond the bare facts.

In Smith's *Dictionary of Greek and Roman Biographies and Mythology* we find it related that Uranos, or Coelus, was the progenitor of all the

Grecian gods. His first children were the Centimanes; his next progeny were the Cyclops, who were imprisoned in Tartarus because of their great strength. This so angered their mother, Gäa, that she incited her next-born children, the Titans, into a rebellion against their father, Uranos.

In the general turmoil that followed Uranos was deposed, and, so that he would be incapable of begetting any more children, Saturnus, the youngest of his sons, with a sickle made from a bright diamond, successfully emasculated poor old Uranos. The records are not clear whether the operation only included the penis, or the scrotum and contents, or whether, like the Turkish or Chinese *taillè à fleur de ventre*, Saturnus made a clean sweep of all the genitals; it is probable that he did, however, as the members fell into the sea, and in the foam caused by the commotion from their contact with the element Venus was born.

Meanwhile, the blood that dripped from the wounded surface caused the Giants, the Furies, and the Melian nymphs to spring into life. Uranos is also represented as being the first king of Atlantis; so that the first eunuch was a god and a king, more unfortunate than any of Doran's heroes, in his *Monarchs Retired from Business*, because he was more effectually retired from business than any monarch that Doran records.

After this the practice seems to have been adopted in a general way; and the fact that the future proceedings of men and things on earth do not much interest these unfortunate members of society in any great degree, interest in worldly affairs and testicles seemingly having been as intimately connected in those early and remote days as with us of the present, it very naturally followed that this disinterestedness, as well as the docility and pliability which emasculation engenders, first suggested their use as servants or in position of trust, as a eunuch, having no incentive either to run away or to embezzle, would naturally be a valued and trusted servant.

In the days of eunuchism there were no defaulting bank, city, or county cashiers—a circumstance which would suggest that such a condition should form one of the qualifications for eligibility to such offices, the very opposition to any such proposal that the class would make showing in itself the benefits that would follow such an innovation, as it would show that the class is not possessed with that total spirit of abnegation requisite in the guardians of public funds.

The requirement might be extended to bank-presidents with benefit, if some Cincinnati episodes are any criterion. It is safe to assume that the bank that could advertise, in connection with its attractive quarterly or semi-annual statement, that the president and cashier were properly attested and vouched-for eunuchs would find in the public such a recognition of the fitness of things that the patronage it would receive would soon compel other banks to follow the example.

The procedure might, with national benefit, be extended as an ordeal to our legislators at the national capitol, as it would do away with the particular influential lobby so graphically described in Mark Twain's *Gilded Age*. These things or ideas are merely thrown out as suggestions to be used by those who write those interesting articles in the *Forum*, or the *North American* or *Fortnightly Reviews*, on government and social reforms, as a perusal of the many articles written in that direction will convince any one that, from a practical psychological view of the matter, they are sadly deficient. To make those articles effective the reflex impressions made by the animal on the psychological and moral nature of man should not be neglected.

Semiramis, whose beauty and many accomplishments, assisted by the murders of several of her husbands by the hand of the succeeding one, had this subject in hand in a far more practical manner than it is generally forced on the understanding; hence we see that she was the first to introduce the use of eunuchs in the capacity of servants as well as in official positions in and about the palace, as well as trusting some of the positions of the highest importance to the class.

From her epoch, eunuchism has become an inseparable attendant on Oriental despotism, and has so continued to the present day. Like yellow fever, phthisis, and some diseases, as well as many other social afflictions and customs, eunuchism does not seem to flourish beyond certain degrees of north and south latitudes—a fact that probably assisted Montesquieu to arrive at the conclusion that climate was a powerful factor in all things.

Bergmann, of Strasburg, quotes the ancient traditions, wherein it is stated that man was taught the art of castration by the brute creation. The hyena is cited as having so instructed man by the habit it exhibited of castrating its infant males in removing the testicles with its teeth, the habit being instigated by a jealousy, for fear of future competition in the exercise of the procreative act on the part of the young males.

Another tradition attributes its origin to the castor. Bergmann here traces out the etymological relation existing between the name of the operation and that of the animal with that of a Greek verb that forms the root of *castrum*, or camp; *casa*, or house; *castigare*, to arrange; from whence also is traced *cosmos*, the world; *kastorio*, the Greek for wishing to build, and the Latin *kasturio* having the same relative but a more imperative signification; *kastor*, signifying as loving to build; *castitiator*, Latin for architect, and *casticheur*, old French for constructor.

The tale or tradition in regard to the self-mutilation inflicted by the castor is traced to the Arabian merchants who purchased the castoreum, which was imported from the shores of the Persian Gulf and from India. It was called, also, by the Arabs, *chuzyalu-l-bahhr*, or testicles from beyond the sea; or, in French, *testicules d'outre mer*.

These terms and the tradition that the castor on being pursued, knowing the reason of the chase, was in the habit of tearing out his testicles and throwing them at his pursuers, were invented by these merchants to heighten the price and value of the article intrinsically, as well as to make it more interesting by this peculiar individuality of adventure.

The Latins, believing and adopting the tradition as a matter of fact, coined the word *castorare*, or doing like the castor. Bergmann uses in this connection a number of terms in French to denote different forms or degrees of this mutilation which have no equivalents in English—for instance, *chatrure*, as applied to animals, making also a distinctive difference between the meaning of the French words *castration* and *chatrement.*

Bergmann is a decided evolutionist as regards circumcision being evolved from prior forms of physical mutilation, as will be more fully explained in the next chapter; the shaving of the head of a conquered people by the Hindoos, or the shearing the royal locks of the ancient Frankish kings; the blinding of one eye of their slaves by the old Scythians, or crippling one foot by the division of a tendon in a captive by the Goths, he considers as on the same line with the idea that led to castration, the different forms of eunuchism, and circumcision.[31]

From a purely materialistic and utilitarian view of the subject, he observes that what we call moral progress and civilization owe their advancement more to material interest and cold, selfish calculation than to any development of the humanitarian sentiments, and that neither morality nor justice has much to do with it.

The evolution of the slave and the marks inflicted upon him by his fellow humans are the most emphatic evidences of the justness of the above proposition. The study of the subject is equally interesting when considered in connection with the evolutions of the Christian Church. In its divergence from Judaism and its beneficent laws, both social and moral, the Christian Church was but illy fit to cope with its

---

[31] Bergmann has gone into this subject at length, and the writer has drawn freely from his brochure on *Castration and Eunuchism,* reprinted from the *Archivio per le Traditione Populaire* of 1883.

persecutors of Pagan tendencies, or to enforce an unwritten law or code of morality or hygiene among an idolatrous, barbarous, and ignorant population such as it had to encounter.

To its professors, the formation of that monachism which has been so much misunderstood and abused was but an inevitable condition.[32]

These men had not the steady compass to guide them in the path that was possessed by the Jewish people. The martyrdom of Christ and many of his apostles, and the teachings of the early church, pointed to physical denials, castigations, humiliations, and sufferings as the only way to salvation; all pleasures were sin and all denials and pain were looked upon as steps to heaven.

The climate pointed to sexual indulgence as the sum of all happiness, as can readily be inferred from the Mohammedan idea of heaven; so, with the early Christians who were born in the same climates, the denials of sexual pleasures were looked upon as the most acceptable offering that man could make to the Deity.

Continence, celibacy, infibulation, and even castration were the conditions looked upon by many of these men as the only means of living a life on earth that would grant them an eternal life in the next. This view of the situation peopled the deserts with a lot of men dwelling in caves and in huts, living on such a scarce diet that they barely existed. That many went insane, and in their frenzy died while roaming in these solitudes, we have ample evidence. The tortures and

---

[32] *The Hermit*, the Rev. Charles Kingsley. See Introduction.

impositions of the Pagan rulers also drove many to this life or death.

Religious mania has caused many cases of self-mutilation, either to escape continued promptings and desires, or simply from a resulting species of insanity. Of the first, Sernin[33] reported to the Medical Society of Paris the case of a young priest who had castrated himself with the blade of a pair of scissors, and who nearly lost his life with the subsequent hæmorrhage.

The writer saw an analogous case on board an American war-vessel, of which Dr. Lyon was surgeon, in the harbor of Havre, in the spring of 1871, the subject being the ship's cobbler, a religious fanatic, who was driven insane by self-imposed continence. We are not surprised, from the lack of intelligence of the times, the extreme but undefined views as to religion that then ruled men, that self-imposed castration should have been sanely considered and carried into effect by Origines and his monks.

The Cybelian priesthood had formerly set the example in their Pagan worship, and when we are told that the monks of Mount Athos accused the monks of the convent of a neighboring island with falling away from grace, because they allowed *hens* to be kept within the convent inclosure, we may well believe that Origines and his monks felt that they were gradually ascending in grace when they submitted to this sacrifice.

As strange as it may sound, self-castration is still practiced by the Skoptsy, a religious sect in Russia. In

---

33 *Dictionaire des Sciences Médicales*, vol. liv, page 570.

justice to the Church, however, it must be said that she neither asked for nor did she sanction these performances, although she was not quick enough in asserting that she recognized the same law in regard to her presbytery that controlled that of the Hebraic priesthood.

Eunuchism presents many contradictory conditions; eunuchs have not always been the fat and sleek attendants on Oriental harems as tradition and custom places them or would have us believe; neither does the loss of virility, in a procreative sense, seem to have always robbed them of their virility in other senses, as we find eunuchs holding the highest offices in the State under the reigns of Alexander, the Ptolemys, Lysimachus, Mithrades, Nero, and Arcadius.

The eunuch Aristonikos, under one of the Ptolemys, and another, Narces, under Justinian, led the armies of their sovereigns. These are, however, exceptional cases; as a rule, the result is as we observe in the domestic animals—loss of spirit, vim, and ambition. The Church recognized this result, and, while the Hebraic law excluded eunuchs from participating in the priesthood as being imperfect and unclean, the Church reproached Origines and his monks and excluded eunuchs from its presbytery on the ground that such beings lack the moral and physical energy requisite in a calling that is supposed to guide or lead men; moreover, there are many reasons for doubting that the ministers of state and the generals of the reigns above mentioned were actually eunuchs in the full acceptance of the word.

Among the ancients there were several methods of performing the operations that made the eunuchs;

some were more effectual than others. From the removal of *all* the genitals, or the penis alone, or the scrotum and testicles, or removing only the testicles, down to compression or to distorting the spermatic vessels, or, as in the case of the Scythians, who often became eunuchs from bareback riding, as Hammond describes a eunuchism manufactured by our southwestern Indians of New Mexico and Arizona, are performances that left many degrees of eunuchism; as we find some eunuchs that not only contracted marriage, but engendered children. Voltaire mentions Kislav-aga, of Constantinople, a *eunuch à outrance*, with neither penis, scrotum, nor anything, who owned a large and select harem.

Montesquieu, in his "Persian Letters," admits this class of marriages as being practiced, but doubts the resulting conjugal felicity, especially on the part of the wife. Potiphar's wife was one of these unfortunate wives; no wonder that she tore Joseph's cloak in her desire.

Juvenal mentions that some eunuchs were held in high esteem by the Roman matrons; it possibly could have been some of this kind of a eunuch that led armies or ruled in the palaces.

Among the sultans and Oriental potentates those who had every exterior evidence of virility removed, so as to be obliged to micturate through the means of a catheter, were considered the safest guards, as well as they were the highest-priced eunuchs, for in their manufacture fully 75 percent of those operated upon died as a result.

It is related that the Caribs made eunuchs of their prisoners of war on the same principle that caponizing is resorted to for our kitchens—the prisoners were easier to fatten and were more tender when cooked. The Italians allowed their children to be eunchized for chorister purposes in church services, their soprano voices after this treatment being simply perfect. It was considered that, in the year prior to the papal ordinance of Pope Clement XVI forbidding the practice or the employment of eunuchs in choirs, four thousand boys, mostly in the neighborhood of Rome, were castrated for chorister purposes.

In China eunuchs were in use during the reign of the Emperor Yen-Wang, in 781 B.C. The Chinese make their eunuchs by a complete ablation of all genitals. In India the followers of Brahma never placed their women in charge of eunuchs. In Italy it was customary to emasculate boys that they might grow up with the faculty of taking the female parts in comedies, their voices thereby assimilating to that of the other sex, this being on the same principle that the *basso-profundos* were infibulated that they might retain their bass.

Eunuchism resulting from an operation owing to disease has at times given queer and unlooked-for results, as, for instance, in the case of the old man that Sprengle mentions, in whom castration did not remove an inordinate sexual desire.

Sir Astley Cooper mentions a case in his *Diseases of the Testes* that is somewhat unique. After castration Sir Astley's patient showed the following results:

> *For nearly the first twelve months he stated that he had emissions 'in coitu', or that he had the sensations of emission; that then*

he had erections and coitus at distant intervals, but without the sensation of emission. After two years he had excretions very rarely and very imperfectly, and they generally ceased immediately upon the attempt at coitus. Ten years after the operation he said he had during the past year been only once connected. Twenty-eight years after the operation he stated that for years he had seldom any excretion, and then that it was imperfect.

In regard to the mortality from castration done in a professional manner and for disease, Curling, in his work on *Diseases of the Testis*, observes that he saw or performed some thirty operations without a death, and that in a table of like operations performed at the Hôtel Dieu, in Paris, it appeared that the mortality was one in four and a quarter.

J. Royes Bell, in the sixth volume of the *International Encyclopædia of Surgery*, has the following in regard to the practice among the Mohammedans in India:

Young boys are brought from their parents, and the entire genitals are removed with a sharp razor. The bleeding is treated by the application of herbs and hot poultices; hæmorrhage kills half the victims, and at times brings the perpetrators of the vile proceeding within the clutches of the law.

The *taillè à fleur de ventre* of the Chinese is a

somewhat primitive procedure. According to Dr. Morache, in his account of China in the *Dic. Ency. des Sciences Médicales*, the operation is as follows:

> *The patient, be he adult or child, is, previous to the operation, well fed for some time. He is then put in a hot water bath. Pressure is exercised on the penis and testes, in order to dull sensibility. The two organs are compressed into one packet, the whole encircled with a silk band, regularly applied from the extremity to the base, until the parts have the appearance of a long sausage. The operator now takes a sharp knife, and with one cut removes the organ from the pubis; an assistant immediately applies to the wound a handful of styptic powder, composed of odoriferous raisins, alum, and dried puffball powder (boletus-powder). The assistant continues the compression till hæmorrhage ceases, adding fresh supplies of the astringent powders; a bandage is added and the patient left to himself. Subsequent hæmorrhage rarely occurs, but obliteration of the canal of the urethra is to be dreaded. If at the end of the third or fourth day the patient does not make water, his life is despaired of. In children the operation succeeds in two out of three cases; in adults, in one-half less. Poverty is the cause which induces adults to allow themselves to be thus mutilated. It is said*

to be difficult to distinguish these last from ordinary Chinese men. Adult-made eunuchs are much sought after, as they present all the attributes of virility without any of its inconvenience.

The study of the evolutionary moves or processes passed by eunuchism in its relation to music and the drama tends to rob these otherwise civilizing and enlightened arts of the aureoles of poetry and gentility with which they have been surrounded.

From Bergmann we learn that the practice originated in the Orient, where female voices were held in higher esteem in singing, and where the profane songs that accompanied the dance were chanted by women.

The Hebraic regulations permitted neither women nor eunuchs to sing in their temples. With the establishment of the early Christian Church in Oriental countries, more or less of the ancient Judaic customs were retained, and in addition a too literal interpretation of the words of St. Paul was adhered to, which said that women should not be *heard* in the Church.

The Oriental Church from these reasons long remained in a quandary; according to the ceremonials, it was deemed requisite to imitate as near as possible the voices of the angelic seraphims, and this could not be done by the rasping bass voices of the well-fed monks; women were out of the question in the then social stage of church evolution; so that at last a compromise was effected by admitting the eunuch, who could chant in a most seraphic soprano, as his prototype, the mendicant priests of Cybele, had done before him.

Constantinople became the centre of learning for Greek music, and the fine soprano solos which now form the attraction of many of our modern churches were sung by the eunuchs. Eunuchs were not only the chief singers, but they cultivated the art into a science, and Constantinople furnished through this class the music-teachers for the world, as we learn that in 1137 the eunuch Manuel and two other singers of his order established a school of music and singing in Smolensk, Russia.

There is no doubt but that in a moral sense, considering that women are generally the pupils, this was a most meet and an appropriate arrangement; for, as St. Alphonsus M. Liquori observed, man was a fool to allow his daughters or female wards to be taught letters by a man, even if that man were a saint, and, as real saints were not to be found outside of heaven, it can well be imagined how much more dangerous it might be to have them taught music and singing by a man not a eunuch—elements which have a recognized special aphrodisiac virtue, as was well known to the ancient Greeks, who only allowed their wives to listen to a certain form of music when they (the husbands) were absent from home.

There is not much room for doubt but that both morality and medicine have too much neglected the study and contemplation of the natural history of man, and relied altogether too much on the efficacy of church regulations and castor-oil and rhubarb.

There are other things to be done besides simply framing moral codes and pouring down mandrake into the stomach; the old conjoined service of priest and doctor should never have been discontinued, as, by dividing duties that are inseparable, much harm has resulted.

Herein dwelt the great benefit of the early practice of medicine among the Greeks, and to the physical understanding and supervision of human nature by the Hebraic law may be said that the creed owes its greatness and stability, and the Hebrew race its sturdy stamina. The wisdom of the Mosaic laws is something that always challenges admiration, the secret being that it did not separate the moral from the physical nature of man. Bain, Maudsley, Spencer, Haeckle, Buckle, Draper, and all our leading sociologists base all their arguments on the intimate relations that exist between the physical surrounding and the physical condition of man and his morality. Churches foolishly ignore all this.

From Constantinople the fashion or custom gradually invaded Italy; and as Rome was the centre of the new religion, so it also became the centre of music, and Rome and Naples were soon the home of the eunuch devoted or immolated to the science of music. The eunuchs reached the height of their renown in music, as well as what might be termed their golden era, with the establishment of the Italian opera, in the seventeenth century.

At this period all the stages of Italy were the scenes of the lyric triumphs of this otherwise unfortunate class, some of whom accumulated vast fortunes. In the following century, as has been seen, Clement XVI abolished the practice as far as the church was concerned, and in the present century the first

Napoleon abolished the practice secularly and socially.

Mankind cannot sufficiently appreciate the benefits it received from the results of the French Revolution; we are too apt to look at that event simply from the unavoidable means which an uneducated class—rendered desperate by long suffering and brutalization under an organized system of oppressive misrule—had adopted to remedy existing evils.

After the dissolution of the Directory France cannot be said to have been in a state of anarchy, and the long and bloody wars with which Napoleon is usually blamed should rather be charged on that government and imbecile ministerial policy that lost to England the American colonies.

The series of battles from Marengo to Waterloo are as much the creation of the cabinet of George III as those from Concord to Yorktown. Waterloo involved more than the simple defeat of Napoleon; it meant the defeat of moral and intellectual progress, as well as the suppression of the rights of man.

The suppression of the Inquisition in Spain, and of eunuchism in Italy; the Code Napoleon; the Imperial highways of France; the construction of its harbors—notably that of Havre; and the political and social emancipation of the Jews in France, Italy, and Germany are monuments to this great man that have not their equals to crown the acts of any other French monarch.

Like the Phrygian monk who leaped into the arena in Rome to separate the maddened gladiators, and who was stoned to death by the angry and brutal mob of spectators whose amusement he stopped, Napoleon's work has had its results, in spite of Waterloo and St.

Helena.

The martyrdom of the poor monk caused an abolishment of the brutal sports of the Colosseum, which henceforth crumbled to pieces. Little did the people look for this result who trampled the monk under foot. Neither did Blucher, debouching on the English left with Bulow's battalions on the evening of Waterloo, foresee, some fifty years later, Prussia extending its hand to make a united Italy, which with Napoleon—who was by blood, nature, instinct, and education an Italian—had been the dream and ambition of his life.

Eunuchism as a punishment is an old practice, as the ancient Egyptians inflicted it at times upon their prisoners of war; so it formed part of their penal code, and we are told that rape was punished by the loss of the virile organ; a like punishment for the same offense was in vogue with the Spaniards and Britons; with the Romans at different times and with the Poles the punishment was castration.

The difficulty of proving the crime, as well as the ease with which the crime could be charged through motives of revenge, spite, or cupidity on innocent persons, should never have allowed this form of punishment to be so generally used as history relates that it was; rape being one of the most complex and intricate of medico-legal subjects, unless we take M. Voltaire's summary and Solomonic judgment, who relates that a queen, who did not wish to listen to a charge of rape made by one person against another, took the scabbard of a sword and, while she kept the open end in motion, asked the accuser to sheath the sword.

Count Raoul Du Bisson, _Dedjaz de l'Abyssinie_, gives some very interesting information in regard to eunuchism in his work entitled *The Women, the Eunuchs, and the Warriors of the Soudan.* Count Bisson has looked on the question from its moral, physical, and demographic stand-points, and, having seen eunuchism in its different aspects, from his landing at Alexandria and Cairo, down through his different expeditions into Arabia, the Soudan, and Abyssinia, his observations are well worth repeating.

From a demographic and statistical view of the subject, its truly Malthusian results become at once shockingly and persistently prominent—not alone in the interference that the condition induces in arresting any further procreation on the part of the unfortunate victim, but in the unparalleled mortality that, in the gross, is made necessary by the results of the operative procedures.

The Soudan alone furnished, according to reliable statistics, some 3,800 eunuchs annually, the material coming from Abyssinia and the neighboring countries, it being gathered by war and kidnapping parties, or by purchase, from among the young male population of those regions. These children are brought to the Soudan frontier and custom duties are there paid for their passage across the border, the duty being about two dollars per head.

At Karthoum they are purchased by pharmacists, apothecaries, and others engaged in the manufacture of eunuchs, who generally perform simple castration; the mortality among these amounts to about 33 percent. These simply castrated eunuchs bring about $200 apiece.

The great eunuch factory of the country, however, is to be found on Mount Ghebel-Eter, at Abou-Gerghè; here a large Coptic monastery exists, where the unfortunate little African children are gathered. The building is a large, square structure, resembling an ancient fortress; on the ground-floor the operating-room is situated, with all the appliances required to perform these horrible operations. The Coptic monks do a thriving business, and furnish Constantinople, Arabia, and Asia Minor with many of their complete, much-sought-for, and expensive eunuchs. They here manufacture both grades—those who are simply castrated and those on whom complete ablation of all organs has been performed, the latter bringing from $750 to $1000 per head, as only the most robust are taken for this operation, which nevertheless, even at the monastery, has a mortality of 90 percent.

The manner of performing the operation is as barbarous and revolting as the nature of the operation itself, and the cruel and ignorant after-treatment is as fully in keeping with the whole. The little, helpless, and unfortunate prisoner or slave is stretched out on an operating-table; his neck is made fast in a collar fastened to the table, and his legs spread apart and the ankles made fast to iron rings; his arms are each held by an assistant.

The operator then seizes the little penis and scrotum and with one sweep of a sharp razor removes all the appendages. The resulting wound necessarily bares the pubic bones and leaves a large, gaping sore that does not heal kindly.

A short bamboo cannula or catheter is then introduced into the urethra, from which it is allowed to project for about two inches, and no attention is paid to any arterial hæmorrhage; the whole wound is simply plastered up with some hæmostatic compound and the little victim is then buried in the warm sand up to his neck, being exposed to the hot, scorching rays of the sun; the sand and soil is tightly packed about his little body so as to prevent any possibility of any movement on the part of the child, perfect immobility being considered by the monks as the main element required to promote a successful result.

It is estimated that 35,000 little Africans are annually sacrificed to produce the Soudanese average quota of its 3800 eunuchs.

When this immense sacrifice of life, the useless barbarity, and the really unnecessary needs of such mutilated humanity existing are fully considered, it would seem as if Christian nations might, with some reason, interfere in this horrible traffic, by the side of which ordinary slavery seems but a trifle.

When we further consider that, in some instances, the child is also made mute by the excision of part of the tongue—as mute or dumb eunuchs are less apt to enter into intrigues, and are therefore higher prized— the barbarity, cruelty, and extremes of inhumanity that these poor children have to suffer cannot be overestimated. Neither must we be astonished at the stolid indifference that is exhibited by the eunuchs in after life to any or all sentiments of humanity, or that they should hold the rest of humanity in continual execration.

Often-occurring accidents in harems make *complete* eunuchs a desideratum. Bisson mentions that on one occasion he saw the chief eunuch of the

Grand Cherif of Mecca—a large, finely-proportioned, powerful black—on his way to Stamboul for trial and sentence; he was heavily chained and well guarded. It appears that the eunuch had only been partly castrated, and that the operation had been performed during infancy; his testicles had not fully descended, so that in the operation the sac was simply obliterated, which gave him the appearance of a eunuch.

In this condition he seemed to have kept a perfect control of himself and passions until made chief eunuch of the Cherif, who possessed a well-assorted harem of choice Circassian, Georgian, and European beauties. The *négligé* toilet of the harem bath and the seductive influence of this terrestrial Koranic seventh heaven was too much for the warm Soudanese blood of the chief; his forays were not suspected until a blonde Circassian houri presented her lord and master, the Cherif, with a suspiciously mulatto-looking son and heir.

A consultation of the Koran failed to explain this discrepancy, and suspicion pointed to the chief eunuch, who was accordingly watched; it was found that he had not only corrupted the fair Circassian, but every inmate of the harem as well. The harem was promptly sacked and drowned and the false eunuch shipped to the Sultan for sentence, the Cherif having the right to sentence and drown the harem, but having no such rights over such a high personage as the chief eunuch.

There are physiological facts and pathological conditions brought forth for our contemplation, while investigating the subject of eunuchism in all its details, that cause us to feel that, after all, the old Hippocratic principle of inductive philosophy, upon which our study and practice of medicine is founded, with rational experience and observation for its corner-stone, is, even if commonplace, the only proper avenue of knowledge.

To exemplify this proposition we have in this particular subject the practical observations and experience of M. Mondat, of Montpellier; in his interesting work on *De la Stérilité de l'Homme et de la Femme*, published in 1840, he details some instructive information on the subject of eunuchs, giving some explanation as to why many simply castrated eunuchs are, like the much-prized eunuchs of the Roman matrons, still able to acquit themselves of the copulative function.

He mentions that while in Turkey he studied the subject in its details, and, having found some of these copulating eunuchs, he secured some of the ejaculated fluid and subjected it to a careful examination. The discharge was lacking the characteristic seminal odor; it was in other respects, to the palpation especially, very much like the seminal fluid.

He found that these eunuchs were much given to venereal enjoyment, but that either legitimate intercourse or masturbation, to which many were addicted, was apt to be followed by a marasmus ending in galloping consumption.

Mondat personally knew the opera-singer Velutti, who died in London; Velutti was, when a child, castrated by his parents, having both testicles removed, being intended by his father, who had himself performed the operation, for the choir of the Papal Chapel at Rome. Velutti was as much of a favorite in his day as our present tenors and handsome actors.

The admiration of the opposite sex was fatal to him; he formed a *liaison* with a young English lady residing in London, and the resulting excesses in which he indulged quickly brought him to his grave. He was passionately fond of women and was able to acquit himself perfectly; at least, as far as the copulative act—barring fecundation—was concerned.

In a previous part of this chapter I have alluded to the very appropriate arrangement which formerly existed when music-teachers were eunuchs, and that our higher circles of society would do well to employ eunuchized coachmen, especially if possessed of susceptible and elopable daughters; but, from the accounts given by Mondat, it would seem that they are not as safe as might at first be imagined.

However, they could not be as dangerous as the chief eunuch of the Grand Cherif of Mecca and increase the population to the same extent; but I should judge that they might be a very demoralizing moral element if introduced into modern society.

If eunuchs must be employed, it can easily be understood why the Turk and Chinese prefer the real, clean-cut article.

The New York *Four Hundred* should make a note of this, as in their present thirst for European aristocratic notions, coats of arms and titles, there is no telling how soon they may cross over into Oriental customs and run a harem, in which case it would be sad to have them make any mistakes in the quality and ability of the eunuch.

Dr. Gardner W. Allen has furnished the American

profession with a faithful translation of the valuable work of Professor Ultzmann on *Sterility and Impotence.* In this, we have a clear and intelligent dissertation that explains the above conditions, and I am only surprised that the observations of Mondat have not developed such explanations before, as the principle was fully explained in practice fifty years ago by the Montpellier physician.

According to Ultzmann, there is a form of fecundating impotence in persons otherwise well provided with an apparent complete apparatus, an impotence which he terms *potentia generandi.*

He states, however, that this form of impotence was not recognized until a few years ago, citing the fact that females have had, as a rule, to bear all of the blame for the unfruitfulness of the family, and that they have been accordingly subjected to all manner of operations, general and local treatment, even to being sent to watering places and sanatoria where red-headed male attendants are employed, to say nothing of the prayers, intercessions, pilgrimages, and novenas to the holy shrines, as mentioned in the chapter on the holy prepuce.

Ultzmann observes that a man may be perfectly able to go through the procreative or, rather, the copulative act, even to the great satisfaction of all parties concerned, and yet be perfectly impotent; he even goes further, by observing that there are cases in which copulation may take place without any fluid whatever being ejaculated. He mentions two such cases at pages 87 and 116 of his book.

In the first instance the ejaculated fluid is precisely as that observed in such cases as those of the eunuchs and of Velutti, mentioned by Mondat, and consisted of an azoöspermic discharge, made up mainly from the secretion of the seminal vesicles, the accessory glands of the urethra, the prostate, and Cowper's glands, as well as the discharge from the secretory glands distributed along the course of the urethral mucous membrane.

Some of the cases of this form of impotence have exhibited wonderful copulating desire and power of endurance, and, even if unfecundating, they must be said to be better off than the victims of that other form of male impotence, the *potentia coeundi* of Ultzmann, where, with a normal semen, either the power of erection or that of ejaculation may be entirely absent.

Peter Charles Remondino

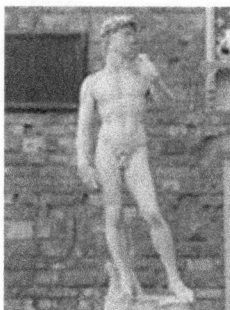

CHAPTER IX—PHILOSOPHICAL CONSIDERATIONS RELATING TO EUNUCHISM AND MEDICINE

Eunuchism does not always subdue the animal passions; this is the view that the church took in connection with the emasculation of Origenes and his monks; the church here held that not only was it possible for them to still sin in heart or imagination, but that, even were the complete eradication of the sexual idea possible, they had by their act lost the main glory of a Christian—that of successfully striving against temptation, and by a force born of triumphant virtue overcome all the wiles of the devil.

It is related that among the eunuchs at Rome there were some who, having been made so late in life, still retained the power of copulation, although the final act of the performance was absent. Montfalcon relates that Cabral reported dissecting a soldier who was hanged for committing a rape, but who on dissection showed not the least trace of testicles, either in the scrotum or abdomen, although the seminal vesicles were filled with some fluid.[34]

Sprengle, in his *History of Medicine*, relates of the complete removal of both testicles from an old man of seventy years of age, on account of inordinate sexual desire, the operation having no perceptible effect in subduing the disease.[35] These cases are analogous to those exceptionable cases in which, after extirpation of the ovaries, both menstruation and fecundation have still taken place.

Modern civilization and its unnatural mode of dressing inflict great harm on men by keeping these parts too warm and constricted. Much of the irritability of these organs, as well as their *decadence* at an age some generation or two before the time when they should still possess all their virile attributes, can be directly attributed to this cause.

A more intelligent way of dressing would result in less moral and physical wreckage, and require less galvanic belts and aphrodisiacs in men under fifty. If those who habitually swath their scrotums in the heavy folds of their flannel shirts, to which are superadded the cotton shirts, drawers, and outer clothes in which civilized man incases himself, would cast a backward eye into the dim and misty past, and see the priest of some of the old Pagan gods soaking the scrotum in hot water, and then gradually rubbing the testicles within, by gentle but firm friction, *to* make the testicles disappear, a process by which many of the heathen priests prepared themselves for the discharge of their sacerdotal duties and the strict

---

[34] *Ibid.*, page 567.
[35] *Ibid.*, page 570.

observance of those rules of chastity and celibacy which they were henceforth to live up to, they would find *one* explanation of why civilized man does not possess that vigor and retain that procreative power into advanced age that was one of the characteristics of our ancient progenitors in the days that breeches were as abbreviated as those now worn by the Sioux Indians.

These are really but leggins, which run only to the perineum and are simply tied by outer points to a strap from each hip. Finely and comfortably cushioned chairs may be a luxury to sit on, but they will have, on the man who uses them in youth and in his prime, a wonderful sedative and moral influence later on, about as effectual as the miniature warm baths for the scrotum and gentle pressure to the testicles that were used by the heathen priests of old, who preferred a gradual disappearance of the glands to the too sudden and summary methods of the Cybelian clergy, who used a piece of shell and an elaborately-performed castration.

According to Paulus Ægineta, this was a common practice of making eunuchs out of young boys in the Orient, the mortality being hardly any; whereas the *taillè à fleur de ventre*, the favorite method for making eunuchs for harem guards and attendants, and more suited to the jealous disposition of the Turk, has a mortality of three out of every four, according to Chardin, and of two out of every three, according to Clot Bey, the chief physician of the Pasha,[36] and of

---

[36] *Cyclopedia of Biblical, Theological, and Ecclesiastical Literature*, vol. iii, page 351.

nine out of ten, according to Bisson.

So prone to reach high offices were intelligent eunuchs that it is related that parents were at times induced to treat their boys in the manner above stated, that they might be on the highway to royal favor, honor, and rank; such is the ennobling tendency of Oriental despotism, polygamy, and harem life. On the same principle Europeans subjected their boys to a like operation to fit them for a chorister life or the stage, where fame and honor and wealth were to be found.

Medicine has been the butt of wits and philosophers, as well as of the men who, from the profession, have gone into the ranks of literature. Smollet, himself a physician, gives us an insight into our wandering and erratic misapplication of our knowledge on therapeutics in *Peregrine Pickle*, where the poor painter, Pallet, is believed to be a victim of hydrophobia. The learned opinion of the doctor, who explains the many and various reasons by which he arrives at his diagnosis, the various physical signs exhibited by the patient as being pathognomonic of the disease, and his final venture with the contents of the *pot de chambre*, as a diagnosis verifier, which he dashes in the patient's face in preference to ordinary water on account of the medicinal virtues contained in urine, which in the case seemed to him to have a peculiar therapeutic value, is something worth reading, however ludicrous it all sounds.

There are few intelligent physicians but who have seen as ridiculous performances, in what might be called medical gymnasts, that equal, if not surpass, those of Smollet's doctor.

Rabelais was also a professional brother, who, equally with Smollet, attempted to waken up the profession by his satires. Smollet was not only a physician, but in his early life had seen some very active and practical work, having participated in and been a witness to the ills and misfortunes that follow any attempts to "lock horns" with nature through ignorance of physical laws and preventive medicine—having been a surgeon's mate in the fleet which assisted the land forces in the murderous and ill-fated Carthagena expedition which cost England so many lives, ignorantly and needlessly sacrificed to ministerial disregard of physical laws and its consequences—lessons which, unfortunately, seem to have but little effect on cabinets, owing to their shifting *personelle*, England following up the disasters of Carthagena with the still greater blunder of the Walcheren expedition, where, out of England's small available physical war material, nearly forty thousand men were either left to fatten the swamps of Walcheren, or to wander through England in after years on the pension-list, physical wrecks and in bodily and financial misery.[37]

Again, the same disregard, born of ignorance and red tape, crippled the British army in the Crimea, causing in its ranks the greatest mortality. It has

---

[37] Smollett gives a good account of the Carthagena expedition in his *Roderick Random*, and for a good satisfactory detail of the blundering Walcheren expedition the reader is referred to Harriet Martineau's *History of England*, vol. i, pages 269, 272, 273, and 354.

seemed as if it would be of advantage if all the blunders, either philosophical or of statesmanship, committed by a cabinet, should be written in large letters of gold, to be hung in the council-halls of the nations, that similar blunders at least might not occur again.

Dumas, in his *History of the Two Centuries* and his *History of the Century of Louis the XIV*, gives some very interesting medical touches. Le Sage, in his *Adventures of Gil Blas*, gives us food for speculating on medical philosophy in connection with the interesting subject of how to make the profession remunerative.

Dickens's ideas of the doctor, as given in his works, are life touches. Witness his description of the little doctor who superintended little David Copperfield's advent into the world, or of Dr. Slammer of the army; they represent his view of the professional character.

Fontenelle, probably, was right in ascribing the fact of his becoming a centenarian, and maintaining a stomach with the force and resistance that are the peculiar characteristics and attributes of a chemical retort, to the fact that when sick it was his practice to throw the doctor's physic out of the window as the doctor went out of the door, as in his day a man required the constitution of a rhinoceros and the stomach of an ostrich, with the external insensibility of a crocodile, to withstand the ordinary doctor of the period and his medications.

Napoleon believed that Baron Larrey was the most virtuous, intelligent, useful, and unselfish man in existence; in fact, it is doubtful if any man of his time commanded from this truly great man so much admiration or respect, either for bravery, courage, intelligence, or activity, as the great and simple-minded Larrey.

As observed by Napoleon of his bravest general—poor Marshal Ney, the bravest of the brave, the rear guard of the grand army, the last man to leave Russian soil—Ney was a lion in action, but a fool in the closet. All his generals had some great distinguishing characteristic, beyond which was a barren waste, a vacuity, but too apparent to a man of Napoleon's discernment.

But the cool, unflinching bravery of Larrey, that did not require the stimulus of the fight or the phrenzy of strife to bring it to the surface and keep it alive; bravery and intelligence alike active under showers of shot and shell or in the thunders of charging squadrons; in the face of infective epidemics or contagiousness, walking about in these scenes in which his own life was as much at stake as that of the meanest soldier, with the same cool exercise of his intelligence that he exhibited in the organization and superintendence of his hospitals in the time of peace; always the same, untiring, unmurmuring, brave, studious, observing, unflinching in his duties, unselfish; whether in the burning sands of Egypt or in the snowy steppes of Russia, in the marshy plains of Italy or in the highlands of Spain, he always found him the same, and his notes and observations, from his first government service on the Newfoundland coast to his last, always showed him the same laborer and student in the field of medicine.

And yet at St. Helena we find Napoleon refusing to take remedies for internal disease whose real nature was unknown, and only toward the end did he consent to take anything, and then only when seeing that the end was approaching, and more from a kindly desire to express his appreciation of the services of his attendants, and not to wound their feelings, than from any hope of assistance.

Napoleon had not neglected the study of medicine any more than he had the study of every other science. This is evident from the instance related as taking place during the march of the grand army from the confines of Poland into Russia, in 1812, when dysentery became very prevalent, of his inviting several of his favorite guard to his own table, where he experimented on each particular grenadier with a specific form of diet, so as to determine its cause and possible remedy. He did not look upon our knowledge of pathology and our skill in diagnosis as being sufficiently advanced or perfect to make him feel but that a treatment for an obscure disease like his own would be pretty much a matter of guess-work.

Charles Reade, in his *Man and Wife*, shows an intimate knowledge of medical science where he philosophizes on the effects of an irregular life and of over-physical training. His logic is sound science.

Defoe and Cervantes show a like intelligent insight as to medicine; and it was not without reason that Sydenham, the English Hippocrates, advised a student of medicine who entered his office as a student to begin the study of medicine by the careful study of *Don Quixote*, remarking that he found it a work of great value, which he still often read. The works of Bacon and of Adam Smith on *Moral Sentiments*; the famous treatise on the *Natural History of Man*, by the Rev. John Adams; the later works of Buckle, Spencer,

Darwin, Draper, Lecky, and other robust wielders of the Anglo-Saxon pen, as well as the works of Montaigne, Montesquieu, La Fontaine, and Voltaire, are all works that the medical man could probably read with more profit than loss of time.

In fact, either Hume, Macaulay, or any philosophical work on history will furnish to the physician additional knowledge of use in his profession. No physician can afford to neglect any study that in any manner adds to his knowledge of the natural history of man, as therein is to be found the foundation of our knowledge as to what constitutes health, and as to what are the causes that lead humanity to diverge from the paths of health into those of physical degeneracy and mental and bodily disease.

We have in medicine many sayings which pass for truisms, which are, after all, misleading. We say, for instance, keep the feet warm and the head cool; this will not always either keep you comfortable or well, as we know that in neuralgias it is absolutely necessary, either for comfort or to get well, to keep the head warm.

While so much stress is laid on the necessity of keeping the head cool, a thing a person is sure to look after whenever the head becomes uncomfortably warm, and to which can be ascribed but few ailments or deaths, we hear comparatively nothing about the thermometric condition of the perineum, which, from the varying temperatures in which it is at times plunged, produces more beginnings for diseases in the future, during youth and our prime, as well as it quite often causes the sudden ending of life in more advanced periods.

People who carefully observe the rule of keeping their heads cool and their feet warm will stand with outspread legs and uplifted coat-tails with their backs to a blazing grate, and then, going outside, incontinently sit down on a stone or iron door-step, or, stepping into a carriage or other vehicle, they sit down on a cold oil-cloth or leather cushion, without the least knowledge of the harm or danger that they are liable to incur. They little dream of the prostatic troubles that lie in wait for the unwary sitter on cold places, ready to pounce upon him like the treacherous Indian lying in ambush—troubles that carry in their train all the battalions of urethral, bladder, kidney disease and derangments, and subsequent blood disorganization, which often begin in a chilled perineum, and, in conjunction with the local disease that may result, end in handing us over to Father Charon for ferriage across the gloomy Styx long before our life's journey is half over.

It is true, neither the savage of Africa or America nor the nomads of Asia are subject to any of these troubles; but with us, hampered with all the benefits of the dress, diet, habits, and luxuries of civilization, and with a civilized prostatic gland, it is quite otherwise.

Herein, again, comes that connection between religion, morality, and medicine, that existed with so much benefit to mankind, but from which we of later days have, in our greater wisdom, seen fit to separate; although, inconsistently as it may seem, the present age has done more than any previous epoch in practically demonstrating the intimate and inseparable relation existing between the physical and moral nature of man. The persistent priapism which oftentimes results from riding with a wet seat and the inordinate morbid sensibility of the sexual organs that may result from the same cause or from spinal irritation are not to be allayed by any homily on morality or on the sanctifying attempts at keeping the animal passions under subjection, any more than will prayers or offerings to all the gods of Olympus restore the eunuchized, either through foolish civilized dress and customs or through excessive indulgence.

We must mix medicine with our religion and make the clergy into physicians, or ordain our physicians into full-fledged clergymen.

The science of medicine, or what might be called the natural ways of nature through its physical laws, is true to itself; the fault lies in our interpretation of its phenomena, which we fail to study with sufficient discriminative precision and nicety.

We have repeatedly mistaken causes and results from this want of close observance and of precision, attributing results to causes which did not exist. As an example, when the early disciples of homoeopathy in ancient Palestine undertook to revive poor, old, withered King David, by putting him to bed with a young and caloric-generating Sunamite maid, when it was by like incontinent practices that he had brought himself to that state of decrepitude, it is plain that they misunderstood the principle.

Boerhaave—who, as a true eclectic practitioner, followed these ancient and Biblical homoeopaths in their practice in a similar case, the subject being an old Dutch burgomaster, whom he sandwiched between a couple of rosy Netherland maids—also failed to grasp the true condition of the nature of things, or the true philosophical explanation.

The exhalations from the aged are by no means an elixir of health or life to the young, and the fact that the young were apt to lose health by sleeping with the aged was wrongly attributed to their loss being the others' gain, and the result of its passing into the bodies of their aged companions, and not to its true cause—the deteriorating influence to which they were subjected; and, further, when we analyze the subject still more, we can understand how a full-blooded and active, lithe-bodied, thin, and active-skinned Sunamite maid might and would impart caloric to King David; but, from our knowledge (not altogether practical) of the difference that exists between differently constitutioned and differently built maids in imparting caloric, and from our knowledge of the physique of the Netherland maids, who are cold and impassive, with a layer of adipose tissue that answers the same purpose as that of the blubber in the whale—that of retaining heat and resisting cold—we can well believe that the poor, shriveled burgomaster could receive but little heat, even when sandwiched between the two; but, on the contrary, he was, in fact, more liable to lose the little he had, unless we look at the subject in another light, and consider that sentiment that is common to both animals and men of spirit, a sentiment that has furnished the subject for more than one canvas in the hands of the true and sympathetic artist, as seen on the awakening and alert attitude of the worn-out and old decrepit war-horse, browsing in an inclosed pasture, as he hears from afar the familiar bugle-notes of his early youth, or some cavalry regiment with prancing steeds and jingling accoutrements, with bright colors and shining arms, going past the pasture, restoring for a time to the stiffening joints and dim eyes the suppleness and fire of bygone times, with visions of gallant charges and prancing reviews; or, how the same sentiment erects once more the bowed and withering frame of the old veteran, and once again fires his soul with the martial zeal of his prime as he sees the passing colors and active-stepping regiment which he followed in the bright sunshine and flush of his youth.

Aside from these sentiments, which might possibly have inspired David and the Dutch burgomaster with an infusion of a new and transient good feeling, it is unquestionable but that some heated brickbats or stove-lids, curocoa jugs or old stone Burton ale-bottles filled with hot-water, would have been more effectual in imparting warmth than either Sunamite or Netherland maids.

It is hard to reconcile the beliefs of some people or nations with their manners and customs. For instance, there is the Turk; when a Jew becomes a Mohammedan he is made to acknowledge that Jesus Christ, the son of Mary, is the expected Messiah, and that none other is to be expected; they know of Christ's speech on the cross, made to the repentant thief; they believe in a heaven full of houris, with large black eyes and faces like the moon at its full, in which all good Moslems are to have continual rejoicings, and yet they go on performing the most barbarous and inhuman forms of castration imaginable, which not only deprives its victims of their virility, but subject more than three-fourths of those operated upon to a painful death, and the remaining to a life of continual misery.

Have these poor subjects no right to future bliss, or in what shape will they reach there? If the heavens of these eunuchisers were like the heaven of Buddhism, or, as the Chinese call it, the Paradise of the West, where, although all forms of sensual gratifications are to be enjoyed, no houris are to be supplied to the saints of Buddhism—as even the women who enter this paradise must first change their sex—we might understand that, the genitals not being needed in the eternal world, it might be considered a matter of small moment to compel a man to go through this short and transient life without them; but where a robust condition of the sexual organs is suggested as one of the heavenly requisites, it would seem as if the Turk would look upon the suffering, misery, and death that they cause, in connection with the inhuman mutilation they inflict, with horror.

Doctrinal theology, whether in the East or West, is something incomprehensible.

Peter Charles Remondino

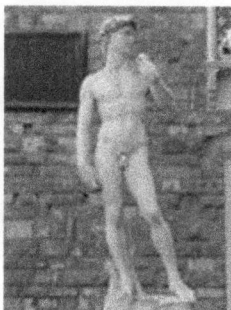

CHAPTER X—HERMAPHRODISM AND HYPOSPADIAS

There exists a class of human beings whose description is connected with the subject of this work. They date back to mythological times, and the confusion incident to the misapplication of names and the want of proper observation on the part of the narrators has tended to carry the uncertainty of their real existence to the present day.

One reason that this part of the subject would be incomplete without their description is on account of the origin of their existence being intimately connected with eunuchism, being, in fact, an outgrowth of this condition; and any history of eunuchism would be but half told, without the additional information concerning these persons.

Hermaphrodites, as stated, date back to mythology. Tradition tells us that Hermaphroditus, a son of Venus and Mercury, was educated by the Naiades dwelling on Mount Ida. At the age of fifteen years, he began his travels; while resting in the cool shades on the woody

154

banks of a fountain and spring near Caira, he was approached by the presiding nymph of the fountain, Talmacis, who, becoming enamored of him, attempted to seduce him.

Hermaphroditus, like Joseph, was the pattern and mirror of continence, and would not be seduced. Talmacis then, like Potiphar's wife, seized on the unlucky pattern of virtue, and prayed to the gods that they should so amalgamate poor Hermaphroditus to her body as to make them one. The prayer was heard on Olympus, and forthwith the two became one, but with the distinctive characteristics of each sex unchanged.

Thus began that fabled race of the *androgynes* of the ancients. Another tradition, which is probably correct, affirms that ancient Carnia, or Halicarnassus, was in those days the Baden-Baden of Asia Minor; that thither repaired all the victims of gluttony, debauchery, and general physical bankruptcy. Its name in ancient Caria denotes its seaside-resort location, Hali-Karnas-Sos meaning literally "Karnassus-by-the-sea," like Boulogne-sur-mer.

The city was under the protection of Hermes and Aphrodite, whose temples were near each other. Human nature in the days of Halicarnassus did not much differ from human nature at Monte Carlo or Baden-Baden. The baths had a number of young and handsome eunuchs who waited on the old, debauched, and nervous wrecks, and the nymph who presided over the whole was Talmakis, a name derived from the salty nature of the springs which fed the baths; this nymph was worshiped as Aphrodite.

Pederasty was one of the practices at these baths.

155

From these conjoined conditions the place was said to be peopled with hermaphrodites—meaning, at first, simply that they were under the protection of Hermes and Aphrodite; and latterly the name was attached to the passive agent in the pederastic art—a name that has followed the class and crossed the ocean into the interior wilds of America, as in Powell's history of the manners and customs of the Omahas, an Indian tribe of the Missouri, we find that they at times practiced pederasty, the passive agent being called by the Indians an hermaphrodite, or double sexed.[38]

The relations that from eunuchism led to pederasty are very easy of explanation. Eunuchism induces an effeminate form, softer body, and prevents the growth of the beard; the voice is softer and more melodious; and their timidity renders them also more effeminate, obedient, and dependent.

The peculiar commingling of the female form with that of the male furnished to the sculptors the models for those wonderfully well-made forms which are yet to be seen, representing in statuary the forms of Androgynes and Hermaphrodites; that of the favorite eunuch of the emperor Adrian being remarkable for the symmetry of its form and grace of pose.

Europe must have been astonished at the tales that were carried back by the early explorers and

---

[38] Schoopanism, or pæderastia, is at times practiced by the Omahas, and the man or boy who suffers as the passive agent is called *min-quga*, or hermaphrodite.—*Third Annual Report of the Bureau of Ethnology.* By J. W. Powell. Washington, 1881, 1882.

voyagers, in relation to the New World. The story of the immensity of the quantity of gold and silver, of great stores of hidden treasures, of the quantities of precious gems and priceless crystals was fully discounted when, from the Florida coast and the explorers of the Lower Mississippi, men returned with the tale that in the everglades and in the trackless forests, intersected by navigable sloughs, there dwelt a people half of whom were hermaphrodites.

Neither the explorers nor their European historiographers seem able to have grasped the true state of affairs. Many believed in the actual existence of such numbers of these monstrosities, while others, arguing from what was then known regarding the extraordinary development of the nymphæ and clitoris, as well as of the great labia, of the women in the African regions, concluded that these supposed *androgynes*, or hermaphrodites, must be women, the dress assumed by these and the menial labors to which they were consigned assisting to favor this opinion.

The early Franciscan missionaries to California found the men who were used for pederasty dressed as women.[39] Hammond mentions the practice as in vogue among the Indians of the southwest, which in a measure greatly resembled that of the ancient

---

[39] When the missionaries first arrived in this region they found men dressed as women and performing women's duties who were kept for unnatural purposes. From their youth up they were treated, instructed, and used as females, and were even frequently publicly married to the chiefs or great men.—Bancroft's works, vol. i, *Native Races*, page 415.

Scythians in its operation, the men being dressed as women, associating with women, and used for pederastic purposes during the orgies of their festivals. These men had previously been eunuchised by a process of continued and persistent onanism, which caused at the end a complete atrophization of the testicle.

In regard to the great number of hermaphrodites observed in Florida and on the Mississippi, the accounts are only reliable as far as they were present in female garb and in an apparent state of slavery, being compelled to do all the menial labor of the villages and camps, besides being used for pederasty, no examination having been made by any traveler.

Their lot was different from those described by Hammond in his work on *Male Impotence*, where the whole transaction seems to have some sort of religious and civil significance. In Florida, however, they tilled the ground, extricated and carried off the dead during a battle, and did all the work generally, being used for beasts of burden and not allowed to cut their hair; but all authorities are silent or in complete ignorance as to whether they had suffered castration.

Pere Lafiteau, however, gives an explanation which was in the last century considered ridiculous, but which, in the light that has been thrown on the existence of a former continent, and of the undisputable relation that must, some ages in the past, have existed between Phoenicia and Central America, seems a strongly probable solution of these customs.

The Father accounts for the presence of these American *androgynes* in the following manner: the Carribeans, or Caribs, were originally a colony from

Carnia; with these colonists was brought over the worship of their Pagan gods of Caria and Phrygia; these two localities were the homes of the Cybelian priesthood, who dressed in female garb, as did the sacrificial priests of the Temple of Venus Urania.

It is true that the Java or Floridian priest had nothing in common with the priests of Cybele or of Venus Urania; but, still, Lafiteau gave as lucid an explanation for the existence of these conditions as any of his contemporaries.

Charlevoix observed the same practices among the Illinois, which he attributed as being due to some principle of religion. The Baron de la Hontan insists that the missionary, Charlevoix, was mistaken; that the persons whom he saw in female attire, whom he took to be men, were not men. Hontan asserts that they were veritable hermaphrodites. The missionaries were, however, correct, as what has since been observed confirms their opinion. M. du Mont, who ascended the Mississippi for a distance of nine hundred leagues, also reported meeting Indians at different places attended by these petticoated androgynes.[40]

As strange as it may seem, many intelligent men were loth to part with their belief in the existence of these double-sexed individuals; the logic used by many of these insisters of hermaphrodism, although now very ridiculous, was no doubt sensible logic one hundred and fifty years ago.

As a matter of curiosity, some of this reasoning will bear repeating. It is taken from a Latin edition of an

---

[40] *Recherches Philosophiques sur les Americains*, tome ii.

159

ancient description of Florida, originally in the English, but translated into the Latin by the geographer, Mercator. In this book we find the roots of some of the myths that led Ponce de Leon and his steel-clad warriors to wander through Florida in a vain search of that spring or fountain of the waters of perpetual youth and of everlasting life which they were never to find. We there learn that, in the days of the good old Spanish knight, the inhabitants of Florida lived to a very old age, and that they did not marry until very late in life, as before that period it was very difficult to determine the sex of the individual.

From what has since been seen among the Indians, the probability is that these were really eunuchs, and probably in slavery, as the result of the fortunes of war, as their great number and servile condition will hardly admit of the belief that they belonged to the same tribe as their masters and oppressors.

Pederasty was an old, very old practice, being mentioned before circumcision; it prevailed among many of the Orientals, and among the many peoples by whom the early Jews were surrounded, who were, according to the Old Testament, about as an immoral, dissolute, and bestial a set as one could well imagine.

Their religions were nothing but a gross mixture of stupid superstition and blind idolatry, pederasty, fornication, and general cussedness. In the then state of the Jewish nation, to have allowed them to mingle freely with these people would have ended in having the Jews adopt all their customs and habits. The aim of the Jewish leaders was to prevent any too free intercourse of their people with these nations, that they might remain uncontaminated even while dwelling near them.

To accomplish this it was necessary to raise a barrier that would be the distinguishing mark of the Jewish nation. Jahns, in his learned work on the *History of the Hebrew Commonwealths,*[41] lays down the idea that circumcision, as well as many articles in their laws—which to us appear trivial—were in reality intended to separate the Jews farther and farther from their idolatrous, bestial, and heathenish neighbors, while at the same time these same ordinances were intended to preserve a constant knowledge of the true and only God, and maintain their moral and physical health.

Although hermaphrodism on a large scale, as an existing condition, was a matter of serious belief at the end of the eighteenth century, it has occupied no little attention in this. Courts have been called to decide on cases to invalidate marriages, or to decide the sex, more than once; and physicians are often asked the question, Do hermaphrodites really exist?

Dr. Debierre, of Lyons, published in 1886 a valuable paper, entitled *Hermaphrodism Before the Civil Code: its Nature, Origin, and Social Consequences,* which was published in the *Archives of Criminal Anthropology* of Lyons, France. In this short but very concise treatise, Debierre gives us a complete review of the subject from mythological times to 1886.

It must be quite evident to all that there exists no logical reasons why the sexual or generative organs

---

[41] *The History of the Hebrew Commonwealth.* From the German of John Jahn, D.D. Page 25. Oxford, 1840.

should be exempt from, at times, being subject to variations from the normal, either through the commingling of two conceptions or of faulty development affecting other parts of the body—conditions that go to form monstrosities.

Debierre gives one peculiar case of a duplication of vagina and uterus in a girl of nineteen, the appearance of the parts and the septum between the vaginæ giving to the whole an appearance precisely similar to that of a double-barreled shot-gun. These monstrosities are as likely to happen as the different forms that affect—either by arrested development or some abnormality of excessive development—the head, which is a very prolific subject of anomalies.

Hermaphrodism is a common attribute in the vegetable kingdom, where fixed habitation or position makes such a condition necessary; it is also common to many of our lower forms of animal life, and even in the human foetus the presence of the Wolfian bodies and the canal of Müller in the same individual attest a primitive case or condition of hermaphrodism.

In other words, humanity begins its existence in a state of hermaphrodism. This condition is found up to the end of the second month of foetal life in the human being, in common with all mammals, as well as all the vertebrates, where, however, it is subject to variations as to time of development and limit of existence in the normal condition.

In the chick, it is only after the fourth day that the genital gland begins to determine whether it will turn into an ovary or a testicle; in the rabbit it is on the fifteenth day, and in the human embryo on the thirtieth day.

Hermaphrodism does not occur, however, from this at first uncertain state of affairs, but rather from subsequent developments of the external organs that by their abnormality of formation simulate one or the other sex, while the internal organs may belong without any equivocation of structure to its definite sex; as it has often happened that some of these cases, having been the subject of differences of opinion among experts during life, were, after death, unanimously assigned to one sex by all of the same experts, the organs readily defining the sex being completely of the one sex.

As observed by Debierre, where the subject is really a female, even where the vagina or uterus is unperceived, the presence of the menstrual function or some physical disturbance at its stated periods are sufficient evidences, as a rule, by which to determine the sex.

The case of Marzo Joseph, or Josephine, reported by Crecchio in 1865, had rudiments of an hypospadic penis ten centimetres in length and a prostate of the male sex, with a vagina 6 centimetres in length and 4 in circumference, ovaries, oviducts, and uterus of the female; it was not until her death, at the age of fifty-six, that her sex was fully determined.

The case reported by Sippel in 1880, supposed to be a male from external evidences, was at death found to be a female. Guttmann reported a like case in 1882. The celebrated case of Michel-Ann Dronart is remarkable; this case was declared a male by Morand Pere and a female by Burghart, as well as by Ferrein; declared asexual or neutral by the Danish surgeon, Kruger; of doubtful sex by Mertrud.

The case of Marie-Madeleine Lefort, to which Debierre devotes four figures, is full of interest. One of the figures is her portrait at the age of sixteen, and another is from her photograph at the age of sixty-five. She has a man's head in every particular of physiognomy and expression, having in the latter figure a full beard and the peculiar intellectual development of a male sage; she has the hairy breast of the man, with the mammary development of the female, and an abnormally-enlarged clitoris, which was often mistaken for the male organ. The vagina at its lower end was narrow, and the urethral aperture opened into it some distance from its outer opening; otherwise she was sexually a perfect woman, and menstruated regularly.

Debierre quotes the case which Duval gives in his work on hermaphrodites, wherein a man asked for a dissolution of marriage, claiming that his wife had a male organ, which, although she was a woman in every other sense, prevented by its interference the consummation of the marriage act. The court had the case examined, when it was found that the erection of the clitoris, which was large, was enough to interfere as the husband had stated. It decreed that the young woman should have the objectionable and interfering member amputated, and on the refusal to have this done the marriage should be dissolved. She refused, and the divorce was consequently granted to the man.

From the history of Marie Lefort, it can well be conceived how the popular mind, in ignorant times, could easily be imposed upon. Montaigne relates the history of a Hungarian soldier who was confined of a well-developed infant while in camp, and of a monk brought to a successful accouchement in the cell of a convent; while Duval reports the case of a priest in Paris who was found to be pregnant with child, who was in consequence imprisoned in the prison of the ecclesiastical court. These cases were strongly females in every sense, but with some male characteristic sufficiently developed, like in the case of Marie Lefort, to allow them to believe themselves men and to pass for such.

On the other hand, males have had some female characteristics so well pronounced that they have passed for females. Debierre mentions a number of cases, to wit: Ambroise Paré reported such a case in his time; Ladowsky, of Reims, reports the case of Marie Goulich, who, up to the age of thirty-three, was believed to be a female, at which time the descent of the testicles removed all doubts as to sex.

Sheghelner and Cheselden have reported analogous cases, and Girand's case—who was happily married to a man with whom he lived until the death of the husband, in which the only female attribute was a blind vagina, which, in his case, seems to have answered all purposes—was a most remarkable case. As a rule, the cases of males who have been mistaken for hermaphrodites have been cases of hypospadic urethræ in a greater or lesser sense of deformity.

Debierre, however, mentions some cases of true hermaphrodism. He quotes a number of cases, the earliest being from the writings of Coelius Rhodigin, who claimed to have seen in Lombardy a case in which the organs of the two sexes were side by side; Ambroise Paré records that in 1426 a pair of twins were born, joined back to back, wherein both were hermaphrodites.

Among the many reporters that he quotes, he mentions Rokitansky, who reported a case in 1869, at Vienna, this being the autopsy of Hohmann, who had two ovaries and oviducts, a rudimentary uterus, and a testicle, with a sperm-duct containing spermatozoa. This individual menstruated regularly, and it is an interesting question as to what the result would have been had some of the spermatic fluid come in contact with some of the ovules that were periodically discharged. Hohmann had an imperforate penis and a bifide scrotum. Ceccherelli, who gives a more minute description of this interesting case, relates that Hohmann, who died at the age of forty, had menstruated regularly to the age of thirty-eight. The penis was imperforate but hypospadic, from whence came the urinary and spermatic discharges, and Hohmann could in turn copulate as either male or female.

Odin is also quoted in relation to the case seen at the Hôtel-Dieu-de-Lyon, during the service of M. Bondet. The subject was aged sixty-three, and named Mathieu Perret. The case greatly resembled that of Hohmann, at the autopsy being found to be double sexed. So that, while most of the cases mentioned are fictitious and only apparent, the fact remains that the existence of true hermaphrodites is indisputable.[42]

If the subject of either apparently or true hermaphrodism is one of unhappiness, and oftentimes of discomfort and misery, history relates that this

---

[42] *L'Hermaphrodite devant le Code Civil.* Par le Docteur Charles Debierre. Bailliére et Fils. Paris, 1886.

unfortunate class has suffered additionally, from the laws and action of ignorant and barbarian times, as such freaks of nature must of necessity have occurred at all times; only in the then ignorant state of medicine and anatomy they must have been considered as occurring much oftener—every deviation from the normal being considered as hermaphroditic.

Opmeyer relates that in excavating in the neighborhood of the capitol in Rome, the laborers discovered the bronze tables on which were inscribed the twenty-two laws of Romulus, termed by many historians *The Double Decalogue of Romulus.* Article XV of this law, as well as Articles IX and X, seem to be directed against the life of these androgynes. In Roman history, however, we have an event which would seem to contradict that there existed any laws in actual force against this unfortunate class. It happened during the existence of the Punic wars, when the people were more or less laboring under fear and excitement, which would readily prepare them to accept any superstitious notion. It was during these times that three of these androgynes were known to exist in Italy.

Titus Livius mentions that the existence of one of these was denounced during the consulships of C. Claudius Nero and of Marcus Livius. Etruscan soothsayers and seers were summoned to Rome, that they might consult the signs and the conditions of the constellations that accompanied the nativity of this hermaphrodite, or androgyne. These impostors, after a careful consultation of all attending circumstances, gave it as their opinion that the occurrence was an unfortunate impurity, and that it could only result to the disadvantage of Rome, unless she at once took steps to purify herself of such a monstrosity, with the conclusion that the androgyne should be first exiled from Roman soil, and then drowned in the depths of the sea. The unfortunate being was accordingly inclosed in a chest and put on board a galley, which put immediately to sea; when the vessel was out of sight of land the chest was thrown into the Mediterranean.[43]

A hermaphrodite born in Umbria during the consulship of Messalus and C. Lucinius was condemned to death, as well as was the one born at Luna during the consulship of L. Matellus and Q. Fabius Maximus. Debierre states that in the reign of Nero this barbarous custom was discontinued, as this emperor admired these freaks of nature from their novelty, as it is related that his chariot was drawn by four hermaphroditic horses.[44]

In connection with hermaphrodism it has been shown that the males who have been supposed to be so malformed were really, in most instances, but cases of hypospadias. It may not be uninteresting to observe that, while during nearly four thousand years circumcision has been practiced without the habit or condition ever having become transmissible or hereditary, hypospadias has shown a decided tendency to being transmitted.

In Virchow's *Archives*, Lesser reports having treated eight subjects during one generation in a

---

[43] *Recherches Philosophiques sur les Americains*, tome ii, page 78.
[44] *L'Hermaphrodite devant le Code Civil*. Debierre.

family. [45] Fodéré records the case of hypospadias reported by Schweikard, in a person of forty-nine years of age, whose urethral orifice was near the junction of the penis and scrotum, but who, nevertheless, had three fine children. The same author records the remarkable case reported by Hunter to the Royal Society of London, also so deformed, who successfully impregnated his wife by receiving the spermatic fluid in a warm spoon and immediately injecting it into the vagina.[46]

Another interesting case is taken from *L'Union Médicale* of August 26, 1856. It instances both the heredity connected with hypospadias and the peculiar circumstances under which impregnation at times takes place; it is reported by Dr. Trexel, of Kremsier, and is as follows:

> *On April 1, 1856, a newborn infant was brought to Dr. Trexel, that he might determine its sex. The father and mother were servants of a peasant. On an examination of the alleged father, he was found to have all the external characters of a male; the urethra, which was rather shorter than ordinary, but of large size, was imperforate; the scrotum was divided into two pouches, each containing a testicle. The apposed surfaces of the scrotal pouches were covered with a red skin, and*

---

[45] *Occidental Medical Times*, Sacramento, Cal., October, 1890, page 543.
[46] *Dictionaire des Sciences Médicales*, vol. xxxi., page 41

the division extended through their entire length. At the root of the penis, in the anterior angle of these pouches, was an opening of the size of a lentil; this was the orifice of the urethra. The lower surface of the penis was grooved from the above-mentioned orifice to the end of the glans. There was no prepuce. Almost in a line behind the corona of the glans, and in the groove, were two elliptical openings, which readily admitted a large hog-bristle; there was a third smaller opening two lines from the orifice of the urethra. This man had always passed for a woman. He lay in the same room with the mother of the child; and they acknowledged having had frequent connection. The woman declared that she had had no commerce with any other man for three years, and the man did not deny this assertion. The idea of cohabitation with another man was further negatived by the circumstance that the infant had the same conformation of the genital organs as the father.

How did fecundation take place? The three openings in the penis were probably the orifices of the excretory ducts of Cowper's glands. But might not these have been the openings of the ejaculatory ducts? It is to be regretted that Dr. Trexel did not examine these canals; their length and direction would have thrown light on the subject. The fact of fecundation may also be explained by supposing that during coition the posterior wall of the vagina supplied the place of the absent floor of the urethra, thus forming a complete canal. This is the most probable explanation.[47]

The above case, as stated, had passed for a woman; these cases are by no means such rarities. The case of Marie Dorothee, mentioned by Debierre in his work, was as peculiar. Hufeland and Marsina had pronounced Marie a woman, while Stark and Martens pronounced her a man, and Metzger could not determine on the sex.

The case of Valmont, noticed by Bouillaud and Manee, is on a par with that of Giraud, in which the party was married as belonging to one sex and where it was not until after death ascertained that the person belonged to the other sex. Valmont had a hypospadic urethra and penis; a scrotum without testicles; ovaries with the Fallopian tubes; a uterus opened into a vagina of two inches in length, which, gradually narrowing, ended in the male urethra, to which was attached a prostate gland. Valmont contracted marriage as a man and was not discovered to have been a female until the autopsy revealed her to be a woman. The relation does not state anything in regard to menstruation; so that her condition in that regard is unknown.[48]

There has also been reported a number of cases in

---

[47] *British and Foreign Medico-Chirurgical Review*, vol. xviii, 1856.

[48] *L'Hermaphrodite devant le Code Civil.* Debierre.

the male analogous to the double organed female mentioned by Debierre. Geoffrey St. Hilare reports a case where the penis was double, one being above the other, urine and semen flowing through both urethras.

Gorè mentioned a like case to the Academy in 1844. Dr. Vanier (Du Havre) records the case reported by Huguier to the Academy, where the organs in the anatomical preparation which he exhibited were so anomalous that it was impossible to decide the sex.

Aside from the medico-legal aspects that these cases present, there is an interesting Jewish theological question connected with them. The law is explicit as to circumcision; the cases presenting, if males, should be circumcised, but how to determine the sex where an autopsy alone will decide the question is not defined.

It has been decided, in such cases where the presumption is that the child is of the male sex, that, like in cases of absence of prepuce, a suppositious circumcision should be performed, so that the covenant should be observed; this being in keeping with the sentiment shown by the Jews when persecuted by the Romans, or, later, by the Spaniards, who often were not able to circumcise until after death; but they never fail to comply with the covenant as far as it is possible.

Cases are liable to occur, however, which, without leaving the question as to sex in doubt, if reasoned by exclusion, would not furnish any possible opportunity for circumcision.

Such a case is reported in Virchow's *Archives*, vol. cxxi, No. 3; also in the *British Medical Journal* of December 6, 1890, and in the *Satellite* for January,

1891. It is one of congenital absence of penis.

> *Dr. Rauber records very briefly the case of a shoe-maker, aged 38, who complained of pain and trouble in the anus. On examining him, Rauber found a well-formed scrotum containing two testicles, each with a vas deferens and spermatic cord, but no trace of a penis. The urethra opened apparently into the anterior wall of the rectum. The man occasionally experienced sexual excitement, followed by an emission into the rectum. The burning pain complained of in the rectum and about the anus was due to the irritation caused by the urine. The man would not allow an ocular inspection of the interior of the rectum. Unfortunately, the details of this very rare condition are incomplete.*

It would be interesting to know where the seat of his sexual desire is situated, unless an aching testicle is such. I once knew a Spiritualist who claimed to feel the pains suffered by any friends with whom he was in sympathy; he once tried to argue with me that a certain lady patient—a warm personal friend of my questioner and a Spiritualist—had ovaritis, because he felt an intense burning pain in his *right ovarian region* whenever he went near to her. I tried to reason with him that that pain should be in his right testicle, but he would insist on having the sympathetic pain in *his* ovarian region.

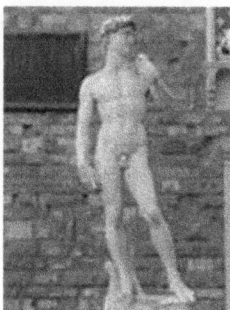

CHAPTER XI—RELIGIO MEDICI

Sir Thomas Browne, in his *Religio Medici*,[49] alludes to the scandal that is generally attached to our profession, we being accused of professing no religion.

That this opinion is still prevalent at the present day is undeniable—philosophers and physicians are believed to be atheists and non-religionists—while, at the same time, by that strange contradiction that is so common, philosophers and physicians are the known and recognized sources of religions, such is the intimate relation existing between physical and moral hygiene.

Confucius, the contemporary of Pythagoras, whose religion was said to be nothing more than the observance of a certain moral and political ethical code, and he who first formulated the text that *one should do unto others as one wishes others to do unto him*, the founder of the Confucian religion, the orthodox religion of China, was a philosopher. Buddha, the founder of the second creed recognized in China, and which

---

[49] Sir Thomas Brown's works, vol. ii, *Religio Medici.*

forms the religion of a great part of eastern Asia, was also a philosopher who was endeavoring to reduce the Brahminical religion to the simple principles of philosophical religion, based on morality.

Moses not only was the greatest philosopher of his time, but also had an insight into medicine that to us of the present day is simply incomprehensible. The Great Master was both a philosopher and a physician, his disputes with the learned and his attention to the sick having given him the titles of Great Master and Divine Healer.

To use the words of the *Religio Medici*, the great body of the medical profession can, without usurpation, assume the name of Christians; for no monk of the desert convents of Asia Minor or religious knight of the middle ages, either in their care of the sick, or giving food and shelter to the weary, or protection of sword and shield to the oppressed pilgrim plodding his way to the Holy Land, were more deserving of the name of Christian than the medical man unwearily and unselfishly practicing his profession.

To the true student of his art there is that in medicine which makes of the physician a practical Christian. Nor is there aught in medicine, either in its traditions, history, study, or practice, that in the lover of his art should ever make him anything but a philosophical and practical religionist. The physician, such as is actively engaged in the daily practice of his profession, instead of having no religion, is really a practical religionist, and, although he may subscribe to no outer ceremonial form or dogma, his life is such that a Confucian, a Buddhist, a Christian, or a Hebrew can behold in him the practitioner of the essence of either of their religions—a conception carried out by Lessing, in his play of *Nathan the Wise,* where the Jew, the Saracen, and Crusader teach the impressive lesson that nobleness is bound by no confession of faith or religion; showing the principle that should guide true religion.

The Rev. Dr. Townsend, of Boston University, has given a very interesting and intelligent relation of the connections that exist between medicine and the Old Testament, in the light of nineteenth-century science.[50] The article in question is interesting in its logical reasons as to why the Bible was inspired by a superior power, as well as in the comparisons it lays before us of the medicine of the Pagans and that of the Bible, during the early history of the world.

After reviewing the false, crude, and senseless vagaries and superstitious notions that passed for medicine from the period of the Trojan war, in 1184 B.C., to the dissolution of the Pythagorean Society, 500 B.C.—periods which existed after the writing of the books of Moses—and the period between 500 B.C. and 320 B.C., or the philosophic era of medicine, during which flourished the father of our present system of medicine, an era of advancement, but which in our eyes is still full of errors and unscientific conclusions.

From these two periods we span over centuries of darkness for science and medicine to the ages of

---

[50] *The Bible and other Ancient Literature in the Nineteenth Century.* L. T. Townsend, D.D. Chautauqua press, 1889. See pages 32-45.

Ambroise Paré and the more modern fathers of our art, who by perseverance finally extricated medicine from the mass of magical and superstitious rubbish which, like barnacles, had clung to it during its passage through the dark and ignorant ages.

After this review our author turns to the Bible and discourses in this wise:

> *Turning our attention to the Bible, we take the position that, though it was not designed to teach the science of medicine, still, whenever by hint, explicit statement, or commandment there is found in it anything relating to medicine, disease, or sanitary regulation, there must be no error; that is, provided the Bible, in an exceptional sense, is God's book. Now, what are the facts in this case? They are these: though the Bible often speaks of disease and remedy, yet the illusions, deceptions, and gross errors of anatomy, physiology, and pathology, as formerly taught, nowhere appear upon its pages. This, it must be acknowledged, is at least singular. But more than this: the various hints and directions of the Bible, its sanitary regulations, the isolation of the sick, the washing, the sprinkling, the external applications, and the various moral and religious injunctions in their bearing upon health are confessed to be in harmony with what is most recent and approved. To be sure, the average old-*

school physician of a century ago would have blandly smiled at our simplicity, had it been suggested to him that his methods would be improved by following Bible hints. 'What did Moses know about medical science?' would have been his reply. But Moses, judged by recent standards, seems to have known much, or, at least, to have written well.

The above statement is a truthful relation of facts, from which it can well be conceived that even in the Bible the physician finds something to inspire him with the idea of its divine inspiration, as the very history of medicine, with which it is connected, and with which he is familiar, only lends him further support in that direction.

Most intelligent physicians are also lovers of philosophical history. None is more entertaining than Rawlinson, either in his *Seven Great Monarchies* or his *Ancient Egypt*. In his *Ancient Religions*, in his concluding remarks, he observes as follows, in regard to the Hebraic religion:

It seems impossible to trace back to any one fundamental conception, to any innate idea, or to any common experience or observation, the various religions which we have been considering. The veiled monotheism of Egypt, the dualism of Persia, the shamanism of Etruria, the pronounced polytheism of India are too contrariant to admit of any one explanation, or to be derivative of one single source.... It is clear that from none of the religions here treated of could the religion of the ancient Hebrews have originated. The Israelite people, at different periods of its history, came and remained for a considerable time under Egyptian, Babylonian, and Persian influence, and there have not been wanting persons of ability who have regarded Judaism as a mere offshoot of the religion of one or the other of these three peoples. But, with the knowledge that we have now obtained of the religions in question, such views have been regarded as untenable, if not henceforth impossible. Judaism stands out from all other ancient religions as a thing sui generis, offering the sharpest contrast to the systems prevalent in the rest of the East, and so entirely different from them in its essence that its origin could not but have been distinct and separate.... The sacred books of the Hebrews cannot possibly have been derived from the sacred writings of any of these nations. No contrast can be greater than that between the Pentateuch and the 'Ritual of the Dead,' unless it be that between the Pentateuch and the Zendavesta, or between the same work and the Vedas.... In most religions the monotheistic idea is most prominent at the first, and gradually becomes obscured, and gives way before a polytheistic corruption....

*Altogether, the theory to which the facts
appear on the whole to point is the
existence of a primitive religion,
communicated to man from without,
whereof monotheism and expiatory
sacrifice were parts, and the gradual
clouding over of this principle everywhere,
unless it were among the Hebrews.*[51]

Medicine is indebted for its advancement to the Hebraic religion to a greater extent than is generally believed.

In the early Christian centuries there existed three great creeds: the Christian, Hebraic, and Mohammedan. The Christian Church was in a perplexing condition.

As observed by Draper,[52] it was impossible to disentangle her from the principles which had, at the beginning, entered into her political organization. For good or evil, right or wrong, her necessity required that she should put herself forth as the possessor of all knowledge within the reach of the human intellect. But the monk and priest were prohibited from studying medicine,[53] as by so doing the church saw that she would have to relinquish the spiritual control of disease were medicine a matter of scientific research; she preferred to hold on to her spiritual dominion, and

---

[51] *The Religions of the Ancient World.* George Rawlinson, M.A. Alden edition of 1885. Page 174.
[52] *The Intellectual Development of Europe.* John W. Draper. Vol. ii, page 113.
[53] *Ibid.* vol. ii, page 122.

let science slumber in darkness.

On the other hand, the Mohammedans, recognizing the principle of fatalism in their religion, it was not to be expected that they should cultivate an art entirely opposed to that principle. In this state of affairs the Jewish physician, led by the teachings of his religion, alone presented the study of medicine in a scientific manner, and its practice and its result taught the Moslems that medical science placed it within the power of man to keep himself out of the grave, when either assailed by disease or laid low by the wounds of war.

The Arabs were not slow to avail themselves of this discovery; and to the learning and skill of the Jewish physician, guided by the light of an intelligent Deity and a liberal religion, does medicine owe the existence of those able and learned Arabian physicians that flourished during the eleventh and twelfth centuries.

There has been more or less of fault-finding in regard to certain rules and ordinances being sacramental, which, from the nature of things, should have been merely advisory or suggestive, as they pertained more to the hygienic welfare of the people than to the spiritual. Thus to reason, is neither philosophical nor in concert with our knowledge of the structure of man, and of the intimate relations that exist between mind and body, or of good health and good morals.

The writer has seen violent catharsis produced by bread pills, after podophyllin, castor-oil, and phosphate of soda in the most generous doses—administered as one would drop a letter in a mail-box—had completely failed; it is all in the manner and way we give a medicine or treat a disease.

Certain narcotic and irritant poisons or powerful sedative agents have a physical action uninfluenced by the mind, but an intelligent physician is hardly supposed to drive at the small tack of disease with such powerful sledge-hammers. Charcot, recognizing the power of and availing himself of such a remedial agent as the pilgrimages to the Notre Dame de Lourdes, is an evidence of the intelligent and enlightened practitioner, who has learned, what the Bible taught, long, long ago, that human nature must be taken as it is found, and that, like the homely saying of Mohammed, as the mountain would not come to him, he must go to the mountain. Moses and all the Scriptural writers were well aware of this state of affairs, and their manner of using their knowledge was adapted and timed to the general intellectual development of the times.

There is one point in connection with the above that should not escape our attention, this being that, while the Hebraic creed and the people still subscribed to the theological doctrine of the origin of disease, in common with the religions then in vogue, here the connection stopped.

All other creeds—not excepting Christianity— looked forward to a theological doctrine of the cure of disease. With the Hebrew, disease was looked upon as the result of some infraction on his part of some of the laws, and the consequent expression of displeasure on the part of the Deity. He was taught, however, that the observance of certain ordinances were both conducive to health and to the prevention of disease, and acceptable to God, as well as to rely upon his study and skill to cure disease.

This was equivalent to teaching them that diseases arose from physical causes, and that physical means were to be used to combat them. From this arose the practice of exposing the sick in public places, that they might receive the benefit of the advice of such who might have had experience in a like case. It is from their religion that Hebraic medicine has received its foundation of intelligent philosophy that carried it in its purity through all ages, free from magic, superstition, and imposture.

With other creeds and religions, medicine, disease, as well as the physical phenomena affecting nature, were believed to be the arbitrary expression of anger of their gods, and that the cure of disease, or alterations in physical phenomena, were to be as arbitrarily effected, regardless of the existence or action of physical laws. It is to be regretted that one of the sects which has sprung from the Hebraic creed, and which worships the same God, has been unable to emancipate itself or its people from the idea of an arbitrary theological doctrine of the origin and control of disease.

It is this creation of a narrow-minded theology of a vaccilating, unintelligent, unphilosophical, and arbitrary God, who would neither respect nor regard the laws of his own creation, that has led the great body of physicians out of the modern churches. They do not deny the existence of the Deity, but the god of their conception is a higher and nobler god—the Deity of Religio Medici.

When the prize for the best essay on the *power, wisdom, and goodness of God, as manifested in creation*—a series of publications known as the Bridgewater Treatises—has been nearly every other time won by physicians, among whom we may mention Sir Charles Bell, Dr. John Kidd, Dr. Peter M. Roget, and Dr. William Prout—not only won on their own merit, but in competition with learned theologians and noted divines—we may truly say that physicians are by no means atheists or agnostics, but that, on the contrary, they are the real exponents of a practical and intelligent religion, which they not only practice, but fully and intelligently comprehend.

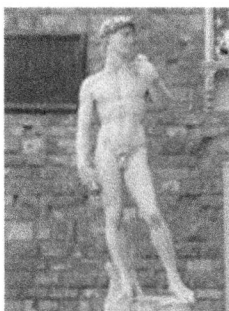

CHAPTER XII—HEBRAIC CIRCUMCISION

The first mention that we meet concerning circumcision is in Genesis. It is the command of God to Abraham; in establishing the covenant with him, He said to him:

> *This is my covenant, which ye shall keep between me and you, and thy seed after thee: every man-child among you shall be circumcised. And ye shall circumcise the flesh of your foreskin; and it shall be a token of the covenant betwixt me and you.*
> *—Gen. xvii, 10, 11*

It was also ordained that this should be extended to servants belonging to Abraham and his seed, as well as to their own children; and that in case of children it should be done on the eighth day after birth.[54]

---

[54] In *Clarke's Commentary*, vol. i, page 113, the reason of choosing the eighth day is given. Circumcision was not only a covenant, but an offering to God; and all born, whether human or animal, were considered unclean previous to the

This was appointed as an ordinance of perpetual obligation on the Hebraic family, and its neglect or omission entailed being cut off from the people (12, 14). In compliance with this ordinance, Abraham, although in his ninety-ninth year, circumcised himself and all his slaves, as well as his son Ishmael. Slaves by purchase were circumcised,[55] as were any strangers, who were also circumcised before being allowed to partake of the passover or to become Jewish citizens.

It was to be observed by all heathens who became converted to the Jewish faith. During the wanderings in the wilderness circumcision was not practiced, but Joshua caused all to be circumcised before they entered the promised land.[56]

---

eighth day. Neither calf, lamb, or kid was offered to God until it was eight days old.
—Lev., xxii, 27.

[55] A father circumcised his children and the master his slaves. In case of neglect the operation was performed by the magistrate. If its neglect was unknown to the magistrate, then it became the duty of the Hebrew, upon arriving of age, to either do it himself or have it done.
—Clarke's Commentary, vol. i, page 113.

[56] Bishop Newton points out the remarkable analogy that marks the Hebrew race as descendants of Isaac and the Arab race as the descendants of Ishmael, from whom sprung the Saracenic people. These are the only two races that have gone on in their purity from their beginning. They intermarry only among themselves and have, alike, the same customs and habits as their fathers. The sculptured faces of the Hebrew on the Babylonian monuments are the same faces that are met in the synagogues of Paris or New York. So with the descendants of Ishmael, in whom there

History of Circumcision

The old Hebrews strictly followed the injunction to circumcise on the eighth day, and of such importance in a religious sense was this rite in their estimation that even when the eighth day fell on the Sabbath the eighth day ordinance was observed. The ordinance, however, was not blindly arbitrary, as rules were laid down for exception. For instance, whenever a family had lost two children through circumcision it did not become obligatory on that family to circumcise the third child, who was however considered as entitled to all the benefits of the congregation or of the Hebraic religion, just the same as if he had been circumcised.

Again, Maimonides, or Moussa Ben Maimon, a celebrated physician and rabbi, born in Cordova in the year 1135 A.D., among his works on medicine, has left directions in regard to circumcision which have been the guides of the *mohels*. Among the Hebraic physicians it was considered that the child partook of the constitutional strength or feebleness of the mother; hence the rule above mentioned, in regard to exemption to circumcision, only was in operation when the two who had formerly died belonged to the same mother as the third one, who would thereby be exempt; but if the two children had belonged to another woman, and this third child of the father was not from the

---

flows partly the blood of the dominant element of ancient Egypt; neither custom, habit, nor physiognomy have changed. In these two races, as observed by Bishop Newton, we have an ocular demonstration of the Divine origin of our faith, if verification of Scripture history is any criterion.
—*Clarke's Commentary*, vol. i, page 111; also, Hosmer's *Story of the Jews*, page 5.

same mother, the rule did not exempt.

The third child of the mother who had previously lost two infants at the rite was, however, to be circumcised when arrived at adult age, provided no further counter-indication occurred. The opinion that the mother gave the constitution to the child was promulgated by Maimonides and became general.

The eighth day is believed to refer to the eighth day after full term; thus, a child born prematurely is not supposed to be circumcised until eight days after it would have reached its full term, and only then if its general good condition is settled.

Maimonides looked upon infantile jaundice, general debility, and marasmus as contra-indications to the performance of the rite; any erysipelatous inflammation, ophthalmia, anæmia, eruption of any kind, fever, tendency to convulsive movements—in fact, any observable departure from normal health should be allowed to pass before performing the rite.

Aside from these general conditions that denoted that the operation was contra-indicated, the local condition of the organ itself also was to be examined, and if certain conditions existed the operation was to be put off. These conditions consisted in any irritation or red appearance of the prepuce, due to either inflammation or to the irritative action of the sebaceous matter underneath the prepuce, the acrid nature of these secretions being at times sufficiently virulent to produce an ulceration, even in the newborn.[57]

---

[57] *Cause Morale de la Circoncision.* Vanier, du Havre. Pages 40-45.

Among the Hebrews themselves there are those who do not look upon circumcision in a favorable light, but on something that has served its time in its own day, and within the past year a proselyte has been accepted into one of the New York synagogues without previous or subsequent circumcision, these reformed Jews looking upon adult circumcision as too painful an operation to be gone through, as they claim, unnecessarily.

It must be said, however, that these persons look upon circumcision purely in a sacramental light, and simply as an arbitrary ordinance of God in the remote ages of antiquity, but which in the present century has not enough practical significance to warrant its performance on the occasion of an adult joining the congregation. These persons look upon it, as has been said, in a purely theological light, and ignore any and all considerations of hygiene in connection with it, claiming that if it is a simple matter of hygiene, then it is not a sacrament, and that, if it is sacramental, then the subject of hygiene has nothing whatever to do with it.

The force of their reasoning and logic is very obscure and clouded, to say the least. The covenant either exists or it does not; to do away with one ordinance in any arbitrary manner is to gradually begin to crumble down the whole fabric of Judaism; for when exceptions are begun, one tenet as well as another is liable to topple over.

If the rite is a sacrament, then it should be performed on all, and a proselyte should not be admitted without being circumcised, and, if a hygienic measure only, the same rule holds. These Jews evidently ignore the rationalism that governed the promulgation of the Mosaic law, and its recognition of the inseparability of the moral from the physical nature of man.

Montaigne has left us a description of the performance of the rite, as witnessed by him in the city of Rome in the sixteenth century. He relates it as follows:

> *On the thirtieth of January was witnessed one of the most ancient ceremonies of religion practiced by mankind, this being the circumcision of the Jews. This is performed at the dwelling, the most commodious chamber being chosen for the occasion. At this particular time, by reason of the incommodity of the house, the rite was performed at the door of the domicile. The godfather sat himself on a table, with a pillow on his lap. The godmother then brought the child, after which she retired. The godfather then undressed the child's lower part so as to expose his person, while the operator and his assistant began to chant hymns. This operation lasts at least a quarter of an hour. The operator may or may not be a rabbi, as it is considered a great blessing to perform this operation; so that it follows that many are found who are anxious to exercise their faculty in this regard, there being a tradition that those who have circumcised a certain number do not suffer putrefaction in their mouth, nor*

does their mouth become food for worms after death; so that it often happens that they make presents of value to the child for the privilege of operating upon it. On the same table on which the godfather is seated all the required instruments and apparatus are placed, while an assistant stands by with a flask of wine and a glass. A warming-pan full of coals is on the floor, at which the operator warms his hands. The child being now ready, with its head toward the godfather, the operator, seizing the member, draws the foreskin toward him with one hand, while with the fingers of the other he pushes back the glans; he then places a silver instrument, which fixes the skin, and which at the same time holds back the glans so that the knife may not cut it. The foreskin is then cut off and buried in the little basin of soil that forms one of the appurtenances to the operation. The operator then tears with his nails the skin which lies on the glans, which he turns back over the body of the member. This seems the hardest and most painful part of the operation, which, however, does not seem dangerous, as in four or five days the wound has healed. The crying of the child resembles that of an infant undergoing baptism. No sooner is the glans uncovered than the operator takes a mouthful of wine; he then places the glans in his mouth and sucks the blood out of it;

this he repeats three times. This done, he applies a powder of dragons' blood, with which he covers up all the wound, the parts being then done up in expressly-cut bandages. He is then given a glass of wine, over which he says some prayers; of this he takes a mouthful, and, after moistening his fingers in the same, he applies the wine three times to the child's mouth. The wine is then sent to the mother and the women, who are in some other apartment, who all take a sip. An assistant then takes a silver instrument, pierced with little holes like a small strainer, which he first applies to the nose of the officiating minister, then to that of the child, and afterward to the nose of the godfather.[58]

The above description of the performance of the rite in the sixteenth century answers to the method of its performance as was witnessed some years ago in France.

In the *Biblical, Theological, and Ecclesiastical Cyclopædia* of Drs. McClintock and Strong the following description of the rite, as taking place in our modern synagogues, is given:

The ceremony of circumcision, as practiced by the Jews in our own times, is thus: If the eighth day happens to be on the Sabbath,

---

[58] *De la Circoncision.* Par le Dr. S. Bernheim. Page 7. Paris, 1889.

the ceremony must be performed on that day, notwithstanding its sanctity.

When a male child is born the godfather is chosen from amongst his relatives or near friends; and if the party is not in circumstances to bear the expenses, which are considerable (for after the ceremony is performed a breakfast is provided, even amongst the poor, in a luxurious manner), it is usual for the poor to get one amongst the richer, who accepts the office, and becomes a godfather. There are also societies formed amongst them for the purpose of defraying the expenses, and every Jew receives the benefit if his child is born in wedlock.

The ceremony is performed in the following manner, in general: The circumciser being provided with a very sharp instrument called the circumcising-knife, plasters, cummin-seeds to dress the wound, proper bandages, etc., the child is brought to the door of the synagogue by the godmother, when the godfather receives it from her and carries it into the synagogue, where a large chair with two seats is placed; the one is for the godfather to sit upon, the other is called the seat of Elijah the Prophet, who is called the angel or messenger of the covenant. As soon as the godfather enters with the child, the congregation say, 'Blessed is he that cometh to be circumcised, and enter into the covenant on the eighth day.' The

193

godfather being seated, and the child placed on a cushion in his lap, the circumciser performs the operation, and, holding the child in his arms, takes a glass of wine into his right hand, and says as follows: 'Blessed be Thou, O Lord our God, King of the Universe, Creator of the fruit of the vine! Blessed art Thou, O Lord our God! who hath sanctified His beloved from the womb, and ordained an ordinance for His kindred, and sealed His descendants with the mark of His holy covenant; therefore, for the merits of this, O living God! Our rock and inheritance, command the deliverance of the beloved of our kindred from the pit, for the sake of the covenant which He hath put in our flesh. Blessed art Thou, O Lord, the Maker of the Covenant! our God, and the God of our fathers! Preserve this child to his father and mother, and his name shall be called in Israel, A, the son of B. Let the father rejoice in those that go forth from his loins, and let his mother be glad in the fruit of her womb, as it is written: "Thy father and mother shall rejoice, and they that begat thee shall be glad."' The father of the child then says the following grace: 'Blessed art Thou, O Lord our God, King of the Universe! who hath sanctified us with His commandments, and commanded us to enter into the covenant of our holy father, Abraham.' The congregation answer: 'As he hath entered into the law, the canopy, and the good and virtuous deeds.[59]

---

[59] *Cyclopedia of Biblical, Theological, and Ecclesiastical Literature*, vol. ii, page 350.

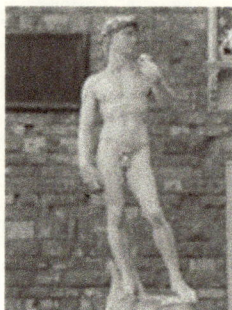

CHAPTER XIII—MEZIZAH, THE FOURTH OR OBJECTIONABLE ACT OF SUCTION

Biblical and rabbinical traditions throw no light on the origin of the details of the operation as now performed. That it was anciently performed with a knife of stone is certain; an event common in its general observance, and which seems to have pervaded all nations or races, howsoever remote or scattered, that it has induced Tylor[60] to ascribe the origin of the rite to the stone age.

---

[60] Among the Semitic race, however, it seems possible to bring forward better evidence than this of an early Stone Age. If we follow one way of translating we find, in two passages of the Old Testament, an account of the use of sharp stones or stone knives for circumcision—Exodus, iv, 25: "And Zipporah took a stone"; and Joshua, v, 2: "At that time Jehovah said to Joshua, Make thee knives of stone." ... The Septuagint altogether favors the opinion that the knives in question were of stone, by reading, in the first place, a stone or pebble, and, in the second, stone knives of sharp-cut stone. These are mentioned again in the remarkable passage which follows the account of the death and burial

of Joshua (Joshua, xxiv, 29, 30)—"And it came to pass, after these things, that Joshua, the son of Nun, the servant of Jehovah, died, being a hundred and ten years old, and they buried him in the border of his inheritance in Timnath Serah, which is in Mount Ephraim, on the north side of the hill of Gaash." Here follows, in the LXX, a passage not in the Hebrew text, which has come down to us: "And there they laid with him in the tomb, wherein they buried him there, the stone knives wherewith he circumcised the children of Israel at the Gilgals, when he led them out of Egypt, as the Lord commanded. And they are there unto this day." The rabbinical law, in connection with this subject, reads as follows: "We may circumcise with anything, even with a flint, with crystal (glass), or with anything that cuts, except with the sharp edge of a reed, because enchanters made use of that, or it may bring on a disease; and it is a precept of the wise men to circumcise with iron, whether in the form of a knife or scissors, but it is customary to use a knife." This mention of the objectionable nature of the reed as a circumcising medium is attributed to the danger that may arise from splinters. The Fiji Islanders use both a rattan knife and a sharp splinter of bamboo in performing circumcision and in cutting the umbilical cord at child-birth. Herodotus mentions the use of stone knives by the Egyptian embalmers. Stone knives were supposed to produce less inflammation than those of bronze or iron, and it was for this reason that the Cybelian priests operated upon themselves with a sherd of Samian ware (Samia testa), as thus avoiding danger. There seems, on the whole, to be a fair case for believing that among the Israelites, as in Arabia, Ethiopia, and Egypt, a ceremonial use of stone instruments long survived the general adoption of metal, and that such observances are to be interpreted as relics of an earlier Stone Age.

197

We are told that when Moses was returning to the land of Egypt he had neglected circumcising his son, and that because of that neglect he nearly lost his son's life; his wife, Zipporah, the daughter of the Midian king and priest, Jethro, seeing the danger and knowing its cause, took her little son Gershom and circumcised him with a stone knife, and offered the foreskin to God as a peace-offering.

Just where the wine was first used we are not told. Wine, however, was an emblem of thanksgiving, and, being one of the fruits of the earth, was considered an acceptable offering to God.

It has since, in some form or other, either as wine or as the representative of either divine or human blood, been used in both the Catholic and Protestant Churches in their ceremonials or vicarious sacrifices, or imitations of old customs. Circumcision was by many connected with a blood sacrifice; it was so suggested by the words of Zipporah at the circumcision of Gershom:

And Zipporah, his Midianitish wife, took up a sharp stone and cut off the foreskin of her son, and cast it at his feet and said, 'Surely a Khathan of blood art thou to me.'

Much speculation has followed the use of this word *Khathan*, which, in the ordinary Arabian, may mean either husband or son-in-law; it also means a newly-

---

—*Researches into the Early History of Mankind.* By Edward B. Tylor. Pages 217-220. London, 1870.

admitted member of a family; a similar word means *to provide a wedding feast,* and one other word from the same root and branch means *to give or receive a daughter in marriage.*

In our own day, the *mohel,* or ministerial circumciser, makes it a practice to draw a little blood from the skin of such as are presented for the rite, but whom nature has not furnished with sufficient foreskin for the operation. The application, thrice repeated, of the blood and wine to the lips of the child, is probably used as a sign of the sealing of the compact.

Wine is mentioned in connection with the High-Priest Melchisedeck as the wine of thanksgiving at his meeting with Abraham; wine was presented to Aaron by the angel, who, giving him a crystal glassful of good wine, said to him:

Aaron, drink of this wine which the Lord sends you as a pledge of good news.

Originally, circumcision must have consisted of the simple removal of the foreskin, and the elaboration of the ceremonial details must have been a subsequent occurrence; persons wounding their fingers will instinctively carry them to their mouth, and it may be that the suction practiced by the Hebrews had its origin in this natural hæmostatic suggestion. Wine as a hæmostatic and as an emblem of thanksgiving and an acceptable offering naturally came in as an accessory.

This practice—which, in the old, patriarchal days of the simple shepherds, when men only lived on the flesh of their own flocks, their diet, however, consisting mostly of cakes of flour, milk, honey, a few herbs, or the flesh of the goat or sheep—could not have been as objectionable as it is at the present day, with blood and secretions in a continued ferment through diet and habits.

Man, living in the open air of Armenia, Palestine, or Arabia, sleeping in the open tents of our Biblical forefathers, living on the simple diet of a shepherd's camp, with the abstemiousness that those climates naturally induce in man, could not help but be healthy. In those early days, when neither passion, anxiety, nor worry disturbed either digestion or sleep, man had no vitiated secretions, wine was then a rarity, and water was the drink.

One of the early patriarchs on such diet would have furnished a dainty and savory dish to the most fastidious cannibal, who is now tormented by the *komerborg kawan*, this being a term used by the Australian cannibals to designate the peculiar nausea that is induced in them when they recklessly eat of white man,[61]—something which they do not experience from feasting on the savages who live on the simple diet of a pastoral tribe.

This primitive gastronomic science in regard to

---

[61] The cannibals of Australia do not eat white people, as the flesh of these produces a nausea, which the flesh of the vegetable-fed blacks does not do. The rice-fed Chinese are considered a treat, and these are slaughtered in great number, ten Chinamen having been served up at one dinner.
—*Among Cannibals*, Carl Lumholtz. Page 273.

cannibalism even reached such a pitch of refinement that, as has been previously mentioned, some tribes even resorted to emasculation to improve the flavor of the animal juices, which by this procedure became less acrid.

The Arabian and Oriental traditions bring us down tales of how, on the same principles, human beings intended to grace the festive platter were fed exclusively on rice. The salivary and buccal secretions, under such a simple diet as that indulged in by our Biblical forefathers, become bland and harmless; not only harmless, but even antiseptic and positively beneficial, acting on the same principle as local applications of pepsin.

So that the practice, at the time of the patriarchs and in their own family, of this part of the rite could not have offered the same objection that it does at the present day. The modern house-dweller, living on a mixed diet and in a climate that induces him to eat grossly, both as to quality and quantity, partaking more or less of vinous, spirituous, or fermented liquors, as well as indulging in tobacco, is quite another being from the Arabian or Armenian shepherd of former days.

Business anxieties and worry also have a very pronounced effect; so that, with the change in the conditions of man and the inception and multiplication of diseased conditions, as well as the creation of constitutional and transmissible diseases, this practice of suction should have been stopped.

Intelligent rabbis, devoted to their religion, are necessarily prone to defend any of the details in its ceremonials that age and practice have sanctioned, and even some of the later writings of Israelism seem to make the mezizah, or suction, a necessary and ceremonial detail. In the *Guimara*, composed in the fifth century, Rabbi Rav Popè uses these words:

> *All operators who fail to use suction, and thereby cause the infant to run any risk, should be destituted of the right to perform the ceremony.*

In the *Mishna* it says,

> *It is permitted on the Sabbath to do all that is necessary to perform circumcision, excision, denudation, and suction.*

The *Mishna* was composed during the second century. The celebrated Maimonides lent it his sanction, as in his work on circumcision he advises suction, to avoid any subsequent danger. Our modern Israelites are supposed, as a rule, to have taken their authority, aside from previous usage and custom, from the *Beth Yosef*, which was written by Joseph Karo, and subsequently annotated by the Rabbi Israel Isserth.

In all of these sanctions, however, there is no reason expressed why it should be performed. [62] Maimonides undoubtedly looked upon this act as having a decided tendency or action in depleting the immediate vessels in the vicinity of the cut surface, and that the consequent constriction in their calibre would prevent any future hæmorrhage. That this is the

---

[62] *Cause Moral de la Circoncision.* Par le Dr. Vanier. Page 266.

natural result of suction is a fact readily understood by any modern physician.

The depletion of the vessel for some distance in its length, with the contraction in the coat that follows, is certainly a better preventive to consequent hæmorrhage than the simple application of any styptic preparation that can only be placed at the mouth of the vessel, but which leaves its calibre intact.

Hot water, or an extreme degree of cold, will answer to produce this contraction and depletion, but there is here a local physical reaction that is more liable to occur than when the contraction has taken place naturally, as when induced by depletion, instead of by the stimulus of either heat or cold. So that if, in the light of modern civilization and changed conditions of mankind, and the existence of diseases which formerly did not exist, we are now convinced that suction is dangerous, we should not judge the ancients too hastily or rashly for having adopted the custom, as it is certainly not without some scientific merit; although, authorities are not wanting who hold that suction or depletion increases the danger of hæmorrhage.

It can be understood that the results of suction would be in some measure analogous to those left by the application of an Esmarch bandage on a limb. The ancients, performing the operation with rude implements and having no hæmostatic remedies or appliances, naturally followed the best means at their command; they evidently feared hæmorrhage, and their rule in regard to exemption shows us that they recognized the existence of hæmorrhagic diathesis or other transmissible peculiarities of constitution.

This same fear of hæmorrhage probably suggested the second step of the operation being performed, as it is by laceration instead of by cutting instruments, showing in this an evident desire to limit the cutting part of the operation to as small a limit as possible.

Against an infant who has decided hæmorrhagic tendency, we are about as helpless as were the ancient Hebrews, and, while the Turkish or some of the Arabian methods of performing the operation may be said in ordinary cases—by the application of cord and the consequent constriction—to limit the danger from subsequent hæmorrhage, still, in the hæmorrhagic diathesis this would not be of any avail; so, as already observed, we must not too rashly judge those old shepherds of the Armenian plains for adopting a practice which to them was calculated to avert subsequent dangers, or their descendants following in their footsteps, until having learned better, even if that practice is to us disgusting, primitive, and useless.

Cases occur—happily not frequently—of alarming and uncontrollable hæmorrhage. The following case is suggestive of the alarming extent and persistence that may attend one of those hæmorrhagic cases, even when recovery eventually takes place. It is reported by Dr. Sannanel in the *Gazetta Toscana delle science medicale e fisiche* of 1844. The case was that of a Jewish infant circumcised on the eighth day.

Some hours after the operation the child was observed to be bleeding; the hæmmorrhage would only cease for a few moments, and then come on with increased force, and which proved rebellious to ordinary remedies. Dr. Sannanel was called during the night of the third day after the operation. A number of physicians had been in attendance, and neither ice, astringents, pressure, nor any usual hæmostatic means had had the least effect; cautery with nitrate of silver, sulphuric acid, and the actual cautery by means of heated iron were tried in succession, without any good results. Ten days passed in this manner, the hæmmorrhage only ceasing for a few moments at a time, and the child was nearly exsanguinated from the continued serous seepage and the paroxysmal hæmorrhages, when a lucky application of caustic potassa almost immediately stopped the hæmorrhage.

This case was seen by nearly all the leading medical men of Leghorn, who lent their aid and counsel to save the little life. The case is interesting from the length of time it persisted, and that even after all the loss of blood and suffering that the little fellow endured he survived.[63]

Dr. Epstein, of Cincinnati, in a letter of March 29, 1872, to the *Israelite* of that city, mentions a nearly fatal case from hæmorrage after the rite of *Milah,* and gives the result of his experience in such cases. He argues that *Hitouch* or *Hitooch* alone, or the first step or cutting off of the prepuce, performed with ordinary care, could hardly be followed up with any more serious results than can be controlled with the application of a little acidulated water. The second act, or *Periah,* the act of laceration, he looks upon as one that calls for coolness, judgment, and skill, as the membrane should only be torn so far and no farther, the thin, inner fold of the prepuce being vascular only in the sulcus back of the corona and at its lower

---

[63] *Ibid.,* page 288.

attachment, where it forms the frenum, or bridle; any carelessness or over-anxiety on the part of the operator in tearing this membrane too far back results in danger of hæmorrhage; especially is this part of the operation liable to be badly done if the inner preputial fold is thick and resisting, as in that case undue force may carry the laceration back into the vascular tissue.

The means suggested by Dr. Epstein to arrest hæmorrhage are those ordinarily used in hæmorrhagic cases, such as will be given presently. The doctor regrets that the operators are not as they should be, physicians, and that, when *mohels* are employed, persons are not sufficiently exacting as to their qualifications.[64]

In France the government has managed to secure more safety in the operation. By a royal decree of date of May 25, 1845, in compliance with a desire expressed by the Hebrew Consistory, it was ordered that no one should exercise the functions of a *mohel* or of *schohet*, without being duly authorized to perform said functions by the Consistory of the Circonscription; and that all *mohels* and *schohets* shall be governed in the exercise of their functions by the Departmental Consistory and the General Consistory. By virtue of this decree a regulation was passed by the Consistories on the 12th of July, 1854, ordering that thereafter circumcision should only be performed in a rational manner, and by a properly qualified person.

Suction was likewise abolished, and the wound directed to be sponged with wine and water. This decree and the resulting regulations have been of the

---

[64] *Cincinnati Clinic,* vol. ii, page 165.

greatest benefit to the French Israelites, and some attention to the matter would not be amiss in the United States.

This reformation has met with the approval of the leading French Jews, whose General Consistory decided that suction was not necessarily a part of the religious rite, and that, as it was undoubtedly introduced into the rite on the days of primitive surgery, it was perfectly rational to suppress this operative accessory, now that that same science, in its enlightenment, pronounced it unsafe.

The whole body of the Congregation did not tamely submit to what they considered an innovation, and from some of the mohels all possible resistance was opposed to prevent the abolishment of this part of the operation from becoming a law. So determined was this opposition in some instances that the Consistory of Paris found it necessary to impose on all the mohels an obligation, bound by an oath, that they would respect the law. Those who refused to take the obligation gave up their vocation.

The Grand Rabbi of Paris, at the time of this reformation, M. Ennery, was one of the most zealous supporters of the new departure. The influence of the French pervaded northward, and the *mezizah* was abolished in Brunswick, Dr. Solomon, a learned Hebrew of that State, being instrumental in having it done legally. The discussion of this subject, in 1845, had one very happy effect—the supporters of the reformed idea of the rite issued a circular letter to all the leading continental surgeons and medical men asking for their opinion on several points in relation thereto, especially, however, on this part of the rite.

The opinions of many of these will be referred to in the medical part of this work.

The after-treatment of the circumcised infant is governed more or less by local habits and the individual intelligence of the mohel and his experience. After turning back the inner fold of the prepuce, the parts are covered with a small, square bandage, with an aperture to admit the passage of the glans. This, and the subsequent small bandage of old linen, which is calculated to hold it in place, are slightly coated with a powder composed of lycopodium, with the slight addition, at times, of Monsel's salts, alum-powder, or some vegetable astringent.

Over these another compress is placed, to prevent the friction of the clothes of the infant or of the bedding. The infant then receives a final benediction, and the godmother then receives the child in her arms and carries it to its cot or crib. The operator generally visits the infant in the afternoon of the operation, and carefully inspects the dressings, to see that no hæmorrhage has supervened.

It is customary to place the child in a bath, either the same evening or on the following morning, the object of this being to remove and to facilitate the removal of the dressings, which are more or less saturated and clotted with blood. After the removal of these, the wound is redressed, as previously, except that some cerate—ointment of roses or some other mild ointment—is used. Some prefer the simple water dressing from beginning to end.

Since the introduction of creasote, acid phénique, and carbolic acid, many mohels are in the practice of washing the parts with water impregnated with one of these before performing the operation, and using subsequently the same form of lotion at every dressing. In case of hæmorrhage there is an hæmostatic water or lotion, which has been long used by the German and Polish mohels with considerable success, and which, in ordinary cases, has been found to be all that was required. This water, called by the French *Mixture d'arguesbusade, Eau vulneraire spiriteuse de Theden,* and by the Germans as *Spritzwasser* and *Schusswasser,* is composed as follows:

Acetic acid, 10 grammes.
Rectified spirits of wine, 5"
Diluted sulphuric acid, 2½"
Clarified honey, 8"

This mixture is well mixed and filtered, and is then kept in a tightly-stoppered vial.

Dr. Bergson uses a mixture composed of diluted sulphuric acid, 1 part; alcohol, 3 parts; honey, 2 parts; and 6 parts of wine vinegar.

Hæmostatic powders are also used by the Hebrews, being more conveniently kept or carried than the hæmostatic waters. In Russia and in Poland they are composed of decomposed or decayed hawthorn-wood powder and lycopodium. That of Berlin is composed of Armenian bole, red clay, dragons' blood, powdered rose-leaves, powdered galls, and powdered subcarbonate of lead.

In France a hæmostatic fluid, composed of dragons' blood digested in turpentine, is in vogue. The Eau de Pagliari is also used; it is composed of a mixture of tincture of benzoin, 8 ounces; powdered alum, 1 pound; and 10 pounds of water, boiled together for six hours, and is considered a powerful styptic.

In addition to these, burnt linen, spiders' webs, starch-powder, powdered alum, and plaster-of-Paris powder are used by different mohels. Touching the bleeding points with a pointed pencil of nitrate of silver is also a practice understood by the Jewish circumcisers.

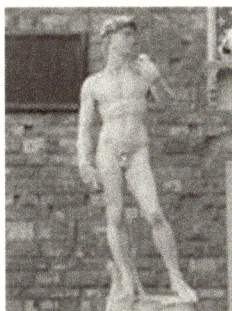

CHAPTER XIV—WHAT ARE THE BENEFITS OF CIRCUMCISION?

There are those, even among the Hebrews, who are so imbued with the purely theological idea of the origin, performance, and causes of circumcision, that they cannot see any moral nor hygienic value in the operation.

Among many Christians the idea still prevails that circumcision is the relic of some barbarous rite, practiced in some epoch away in the remote ages of the world, grafted on to the Jewish religion by some accident or other; but that beyond the clinging of the Jews to this custom, as being a remnant of their old religion, they neither see in the rite any other significance, moral results, nor hygienic precaution; and the fact of a Jew being circumcised is too often made a subject of merriment among the unthinking portion of the Christian world.

Neither are physicians all of one accord on the subject as to whether circumcision is a benefit, or, being useless, a dangerous and an unnecessary operation. The writer is most emphatically in favor of circumcision, and has the fullest faith in the positive moral and physical benefits that mankind gains from the operation.

It may well be asked: what does the Jew receive in return for all the suffering that he inflicts through circumcision on himself and his little children? What is there to repay him or his for all the risks and annoyances, besides branding himself and his with an indestructible mark, which has been more than once the sign by which they have suffered persecution, spoliation, expatriation, and death? Are there any benefits enjoyed by the Jew that the uncircumcised does not enjoy in equal proportion?

The relative longevity between the Hebrew race and the Christian nations that dwell together under like climatic and political conditions indicates a stronger tenacity on the part of the Jewish part of the nations to life, a greatly less liability to disease, and a stronger resistance to epidemic, endemic, and accidental diseases.

By some authorities it has been held that the occupations followed by the Jew are such as do not compel him to risk his life, as he neither follows any labor requiring any great and continued exertion, nor any that subjects him to any great exposure; that, as a rule, when in business, by some intuition he follows some branch that has neither anxiety, care, nor great chance of loss connected with it; that he does not follow any occupation that is attended with any risk of accident for either life or limb.

Besides all these, it is also urged that in cities the careful inspection of their meat, and the peculiar social fabric of the family, the love and veneration for their aged, as well as their proverbial charity to their own poor and sick, and their provident habits and hygienic regulations imposed upon them by the Mosaic law, are all conditions that conspire to induce longevity.

That the Hebrew is generally found in such conditions as above described is undisputed; but it is questionable if all these conditions are necessarily such as are favorable to health and long life, and that, therefore, the longevity of the Jewish race cannot altogether be ascribed to the above conditions.

Looking at the subject of occupation, if we consult Lombard, Thackrah, and the later works on the effects of occupation on life, we must admit that the Jew has no visible advantage in that regard, as he follows hardly any out-of-door occupation, being often indoors in a confined and foul atmosphere. To those who have closely observed the race in this country—coming as they do from the cold-wintered climates of Germany, Austria, or Poland, bringing with them the habit of living in small, close rooms, for the sake of economy and comfort—it must be admitted that among the lower classes and the poorer of the race, their shops being connected, as they usually are, with their living-rooms, the *toute ensemble* is anything but conducive to a long life.

Their anæmic and undeveloped physical condition and weak muscular organization are sufficient evidence that their surroundings are not calculated to improve health. In England, statistics sufficiently prove that the fisherman on the coast, exposed to all kinds of weather, is not as prone to disease as is his brother Englishman who deals out the groceries in his snug shop. Exercise has been held an important element in the factory of the long-lived. From the time of Hippocrates down to Cheyne, Rush, Hufeland, Tissot, Charcot, Humphry, and all authorities on the factors of old age, exercise has been looked upon as favoring long life.

Exercise cannot be said to enter in any way as a factor in the longevity of the Jew; but, on the contrary, his in-door life is known to be very productive of phthisis in other races. His recreations are, as a rule, of the home social order. They visit and spend the time allotted to recreation in social intercourse, which their hospitality always insists on accompanying with a generous lunch, which, to say the least, is not an element that is conducive to either health or long life; for no people excel the Jew in home hospitality, and even among the poorer classes a stranger is never allowed to depart without some refreshment being offered him.

Among the class better able to extend hospitality, social reunions and card parties, with lunches of fruits, cakes, cold meats and coffee, or wines, are among their regular occurrences. Their great affection for the family and for their youth and aged suggests these means of recreation, as then they are enjoyed by all alike; but, as observed, the hygiene of all this is very doubtful; it produces too much irregularity.

It is related that after the Roman conquest of Palestine many of the Jews, becoming more or less accustomed to Roman manners and customs, often joined in the games which the Romans held in imitation of the old Olympic games of the Grecians.

History of Circumcision

Not to be ridiculed, many resorted to the practices described in a previous chapter, to efface all the marks of their circumcision, that they might enter the games with as much freedom as the Romans or other uncircumcised nations; so that the present aversion to out-of-door sports evinced by the Jew is not necessarily a racial trait; the persecutions and political inequality that until lately he has been made to suffer have driven him into retirement and seclusion.

Although seeking neither converts nor political power and influence, he has been hunted down, massacred, and chased about as a dangerous beast. As the children of the great Rabbi Moses Mendelssohn asked of their father:

Is it a disgrace to be a Jew? Why do people throw stones at us and call us names?

It may well be asked, why? These actions have forced them into the social and retired habits for which they are noted; although it cannot be said that it is from a lack of spirit, as one of the Rothschilds is well known to have been present at the battle of Waterloo, where from a spot in the vicinity of the British right-centre he observed the events of the battle; and when, with the failure of Ney's last desperate charge with the formidable battalions of the Old Guard, he saw the advance of the Prussians closing in on the French right, he galloped to the sea-shore, and, crossing the Channel in a frail boat, reached London twenty-four hours in advance of the news of the battle,[65] but long

---

[65] *The Story of the Jews*, Hosmer. Page 263.

enough for him to clear several millions from off the panicky state of the money market.

Marshal Massena, one of Napoleon's bravest generals, the defender of Genoa and the hero of Wagram, was of Jewish origin.

Athletic sports are not of necessity conducive to long life, even if they are to temporary robust health; but there is no mistaking the fact that the sedentary and in-door life of the average Jew is a deteriorator to health and life, and especially among that class of families who are poor and keep no servant; from heredity and home education having adopted unhygienic customs, in which they have grown up—in these a total disregard for all ventilation forms a part.

Were an uncircumcised race so to live, scrofula and phthisis would be the inevitable result. This difference of results I have witnessed more than once as existing among the two races coming from the same European nationality, where their disregard to ordinary rules of hygiene, induced by climatic causes, especially ventilation, were alike in both the Semitic and European descendants of the one nation, the purely European being more prone to consumption and scrofula.

It is interesting to note the difference in the moral, mental, and physical conditions induced by creeds; it would seem as if it should not make any difference. The generally accepted idea of religion is that it should raise the moral standard of all those nations who practice religion; but the results are very peculiar, as we are forced to admit that reformation in religion has not always been a reformation in morals. Take Great Britain for example; if illegitimacy is any criterion of the moral state of those professing creeds, we find the least among the Jew; next among the Catholic; next comes the Episcopalian; then last the Presbyterian— the oldest creed showing the greatest moral tendency, and that of poor Knox, which is the youngest, showing the least. This has certainly its physical effects, that are not without its influence in producing a greater or lesser length of life. The evolution of religion has here induced a lower moral tone and a resulting physical degeneracy.

As observed by alienists, religions of different creeds have different tendencies in inducing insanity, both as to ratio of population and as to manifestations;[66] the Protestant, when unbalanced by religious cause, is generally controlled with some idea that shows itself in wild and erratic attempts at scriptural interpretation, caused by want of fixed dogmas and the unending splittings that are forever taking place in the new faith, and the persistent, intrusive, and belligerent spirit of proselytism that controls each new branch as it buds into existence.

The Catholic has a fixed dogma, which the church attends to, and he neither feels called upon to make his neighbors miserable or himself insane in hunting up new interpretations. When he does go insane on the subject of religion, the cause, as a rule, can be traced to some real or imagined moral delinquency, which has brought all the terrors of the punishment of the damned forcibly and persistently to his disordered imagination.

---

66 *Traité d'Hygiène*, publique et privée, Michel Levy. 2d. edition, vol. ii, page 754.

Peter Charles Remondino

In the insane-asylums of Cork, in Ireland, with its overwhelming Catholic population, the ratio of inmates in regard to creeds is as that of one Catholic to ten of the Reformed religion, showing in the most conclusive manner the influence exerted by religion in this direction.

On the other hand, the Jew has the simplest of religious creeds; he neither wastes useful time, robs himself of sleep, nor becomes dyspeptic in hunting for hidden meanings in some ambiguous scriptural phrase; he is satisfied with his creed, his dogmas are firmly anchored, and the nature of his religion being a sort of family congregation, he is not called upon to go out in search of proselytes, any more than the father of an already large family feels called upon to go out and hunt up the homeless, that he may convert his home into a promiscuous orphan-asylum.

As before remarked, his creed is of the simplest, and there exists a complete and explicit understanding between his God and himself. There are no mystical, hidden meanings in Scripture for the Jew; nor does he dread any eternal, unheard-of, and inexplicable torments. His laws are very clear, and the punishments for their infraction very explicit. To the Jew it is a straight and well-lighted road, as far as religion is concerned.

The writer has always felt that it took a mind that was incapable of appreciating simple truths, but that loved to hover on that mystical border-land on the confines of gloomy insanity that would allow its owner to seriously wander through and behold any theological beauties in Bunyan.

To the Jew there is none of the gloomy, weird,

218

mystical, mind-racking, ungodly theology that some of our creeds torture the poor brains of their professors with. As the wild Indian of the plains runs sticks through his anatomy and capers wildly about to torture his body, so some of the creeds delight in torturing their devotees.

The Jewish religion is the one best suited to tranquilize the mind; it is very philosophical and rational. Were he to acknowledge Christ, he would not have to change his course of life to become a most exemplary Christian. The celebrated letter of Moses Mendelssohn to the Swiss clergyman, Lavater, in answer to a dedication of the latter to Mendelssohn, is probably the best exposition of the essence of the Jewish faith that can be found. Therein he says:

We believe that all other nations of the earth have been commanded by God to adhere to the laws of nature. Those who regulate their conduct according to this religion of nature and of reason are called virtuous men of other nations, and are the children of eternal salvation.

Such a religion does not unsettle man's mind.

These apparent digressions are made to show what additional factors exist, besides circumcision, to induce longevity in the Jewish race, and that the subject may be better understood; for these reasons the above comparisons have been made. Students of demographic science are well aware that form of government, religion, climate, diet, habit, and custom—all have an important bearing on the mental and physical as well as on the moral nature of man.

To the true student of his art all these conditions are but factors in the physical scale, and should so be considered without fear or favor; to him the whole world is but a unit, and the people upon its surface are but as one people, alike subject to the leveling laws of nature, which recognize neither royalty nor vagrant, nationality nor creed, color, condition, nor station in life or society.

Professor Bernoulli, of Bale, found the Israelite less prolific than the Christian;[67] subject to less mortality, greater longevity, less still-born, less illegitimacy, less crime against the person, and less insanity and suicide, when compared with his Christian brother— all of which he attributes not to a superior physique or organism, but solely to the observance of the laws of their religion and to the nature of the same, which exercises a beneficial influence on the mind.

B. W. Richardson, in his *Diseases of Modern Life*, in speaking of the relation of race to disease, says:

> *Through the valuable labors of MM. Legoyt, Hoffmann, Neufville, and Mayer, we have obtained, however, some curious facts relative to the most widely disseminated of all races on the earth, the Jewish. These facts show that, from some cause or causes, this race presents an endurance against disease that does not belong to other portions of the civilized communities amongst which its members dwell. The*

---

[67] *Ibid.*

distinctness of the Jews in the midst of other and mixed races singles them out specially for observation, and the history they present of vitality, or, in other words, of the resistance to those influences which tend to shorten the natural cycle of life, is singularly instructive.

The resistance dates from the first to the last periods of life. Hoffmann finds that in Germany, from 1823 to 1840, the number of still-born among the Jews was as 1 in 39, while with other races it was 1 in 40. Mayer finds that in Furth children from one to five years of age die in the proportion of 10 per cent. among the Jewish, and 14 per cent. among the Christian population. M. Neufville, dealing with the same subject, from the statistics of Frankfurt, gives even a more favorable proportion of vitality to the Jewish child population. Continuing his estimates from the ages named into riper years, the value of life is still in favor of the Jews, the average duration of the life of the Jew being forty years and nine months and that of the Christian being thirty-six years and eleven months. In the total of all ages, the half of the Jews born reach the age of fifty-three years and one month, whilst half of the Christians born only reach the age of thirty-six years. A quarter of the Jewish population born is found living beyond seventy-one years, but a quarter of the Christian population is found living beyond fifty-nine years and ten months only. The Civil State extracts of Prussia give to the Jews a mortality of 1.61 per cent.; to the whole kingdom, 2.62 per cent. To the Jews they give an annual increase of 1.73 per cent.; to the Christian, 1.36 per cent. The effective of the Jews require a period of forty-one years and a half to double themselves; those of other races, fifty-one years. In 1849, Prussia returned one death for every forty-one of the Jews and one for every thirty-two of the remaining population. The Jews escaped the great epidemics more readily than the other races with whom they lived. Thus, the mortality from cholera amongst them is so small that the very fact of its occurrence has been disputed. Lastly, that element of mortality, suicide, which we may look upon philosophically as a phenomenon of disease, is computed by Glatter, from a proportion of one million of inhabitants of Prussia, Bavaria, Würtemburg, Austria, Hungary, and Transylvania, to have been committed by rather less than one of the Jewish race to four of the members of the mixed races of the Christian population. Different causes have been assigned for this higher vitality of the Jewish race, and it were indeed wise to seek for the causes, since that race which presents the strongest vitality, the greatest increase of life, and the longest resistance to death must in course of time become, under the influences of civilization, dominant. We see this truth, indeed, actually exemplified in the Jews; for no other known race has ever endured so much or resisted so much. Persecuted, oppressed by every imaginable form of tyranny, they have held together and lived, carrying on intact their customs, their beliefs, their faith, for centuries, until, set free at last, they flourish as if endowed with new force. They rule more potently than ever, far more potently than when Solomon in all his glory reigned in Jerusalem. They rule, and neither fight nor waste.[68]

Richardson attributes the great benefits enjoyed in this regard by the Jewish race to the soberness of their lives.

This position is, however, not altogether tenable, if by that we mean abstemiousness; they are extremely temperate, but not abstemious. Tissot, Cornaro, Lessius, Hufeland, Humphry, Sir Henry Thompson, as well as the older Greek and Roman authorities, all are agreed that an abstemious life is the one that is most conducive to long life.

There is no race that is more proverbial for their good cheer and indulgence in the good things of the table than the Jewish; no race enjoys feasting any more than they, and from childhood they are accustomed to a generous and nutritious diet, as well

---

[68] *Diseases of Modern Life.* B. W. Richardson. Page 19.

as to their share of the wines with which their tables are supplied.

Their greater thrift and application to business, their habits of economy and carefulness in business affairs enable them to better supply their tables. In California there is no class that lives better or whose tables are supplied so well either as to quality or quantity as those of the Jews, and yet no class is more exempt than they from the class of diseases that originate in too good living.

As before remarked, in relation to the poor of that faith, who are unable to keep a servant, and who live in a combination of shop and home in the most unhygienic condition, disregarding ventilation and every other sanitary needs, but who, nevertheless, escape the evil results that would and do attend such social conditions among those of other races, so in this instance of good living: the better class of Jews do not suffer in anything near a like proportion to the better class Christians from diseases incident to too full habits and an inactive life.

Richardson observes that he drinks less and that he eats better food than his Christian brother. In regard to the drinking habit, overindulgence is not a Jewish failing; they do not drink to excess, but total abstinence is not in their vocabulary. It is inconsistent with their idea of wine as being a gift of God, and something that is symbolical of good faith and thanksgiving.

Nor is total abstinence consistent with their idea of generous hospitality. On the eighth day after birth the Jew tastes wine, and from the time he is able to sit at table he becomes familiar with its use. To him wine is not symbolical of either moral depravity, mental or physical deterioration, or of death.

Their females are all accustomed to its use from childhood, but it does not cause them to become either immoral or unchaste; so that in neither sex does wine produce that moral and mental wreckage which abbreviates the length of human existence among those of other creeds. Radical fanaticism, that drives a tack with a maul and a twenty-penny spike with a tack-hammer, cannot be expected to study this or any other question in any rational manner; but to the sociologist, the question as to what produces this remarkable soberness, in the midst of the habitual and continued use of wine in the race from the time of its earliest history, is something worthy of calm and careful consideration.

How much circumcision may have to do with this will be discussed in the medical part of the volume.

In London, according to Dr. Stallard, the mortality among Jewish children from one to five years is only ten percent, while among the children of the Christians it is fourteen percent, the rate being analogous to that observed by Mayer among those of these ages in Furth. Among the London adults the average duration of life among the Jews is forty-seven years, while among the Christians it is only thirty-seven.

Dr. Hough [69] has gathered some interesting historical and statistical matter bearing on the subject

---

[69] *Longevity and other Biostatic Peculiarities of the Jewish Race.* By John Stockton Hough, M.D. *New York Med. Record,* 1873.

of Jewish resistance to disease and the benefit possessed by the race in relation to the immunity enjoyed by them in prevailing epidemics.

The plague of 1346 did not affect them; according to Fracastor they escaped the typhus of 1505; Rau remarks their immunity to the typhus of 1824; Ramazzini noticed their exemption to the fatal intermittents of Rome, in 1691; and Degner says that they escaped the epidemic dysentery at Nimegue, in 1736. Richardson truly observes that

> ...*from epidemics the Jews have often escaped, as if they possessed a charmed life.*

This racial difference and benefit, when compared to other races, has more than once cost them dear. In the dark and ignorant ages, when men reasoned nothing from a physical basis, but attributed all and every phenomena to some supernatural agency, either heavenly or diabolical, it was but natural for such minds to associate this exemption with some purchased compact made with the devil, who was often also held accountable for the existence of the epidemics.

The rational and law-of-nature observing Jew supposed to be in league with his satanic majesty could neither be seen nor heard in his own defense; consequently, massacres, pillaging, and such other barbarities that an insane popular fury could suggest, were the humane manifestations with which a Christian people visited their Jewish brothers, whose only sin consisted in worshiping the God of their fathers, and in strictly observing His laws and commandments.

In France, Dr. Neufville found that, of one hundred children in the first five years of life, among the Jewish population, 12.9 die; while from the same number of the same aged class of Christians 24.1 die. One-half of all the Christians die at thirty-six years, and one-half of all the Jews at fifty-three years and one month.

Dr. John S. Billings has gathered statistics relating to 10,618 Jewish families, consisting of 60,630 persons,[70] living in the United States in December, 1889, mostly descendants of Jews from the northern or middle nations of Europe.

For our purpose only the deductions as to death-rate and tendency to longevity will be given. In this valuable paper Dr. Billings says:

> *When we come to examine the reports of deaths for five years furnished by these Jewish families, we find that they give an average annual death-rate of only 7.1 per 1000, which would be about one-half of the annual death-rate among other persons of the same average social class and condition living in this country.*

To this he adds that, provided the deaths at different ages among the Jews have been correctly reported, this race will, on comparison with those of other races, show a greater tendency to longevity, as the Jewish

---

[70] *Vital Statistics of the Jews*, Dr. John S. Billings. *North American Review*, No. 1, vol. 152, page 70, January, 1891.

expectation of life is at each age markedly greater than that of the class of people who insure their lives, the average excess being a little over twenty per cent.

In speaking of the death-rate among children, Dr. Billings makes the following comparisons:

> *The low death-rate among the Jews is especially marked among the children, and this corresponds to European experience. Thus in Prussia, in 1887, the death-rate of the Jews under fifteen years of age was 5.63 for 1000, while among the remainder of the people it was 10.46 per 1000.*

This result he accounts for partly to the fact that among the Jews illegitimacy is comparatively rare and to the high rate of mortality among the illegitimate born, which raises the average of the other classes.

In regard to the immunity of the race from consumption or tubercular disease, the statistics of the above Jewish families gives to the Jews less than one-third of the number of deaths from these diseases than what occurs among the others as to the male population, and less than one-fourth as to the female population.

These statistics coincide with the observations of the writer on this part of the subject, and are even more than corroborated by the French War-Office Reports from Algeria, where the deaths from consumption among the Christians amount to 1 for each 9.3 deaths, and among the Jews to 1 in 36.9, while among the Mohammedans it is only 1 in 40.7 deaths.

In Algeria the relative mortality from all causes is only about three-fifths of that of the Christian, and the Turk, although seeming to enjoy a greater exemption from phthisical or tubercular diseases than the Jew, falls below the Jew in exemption from deaths due to general causes, as his mortality is one-eighth greater than that of the Jew.

Dr. Billings gives us some interesting food for thought in the course of his article and some more particularly bearing on the subject of immunity from consumption. He asks:

> *Are these differences due to race characteristics, properly so-called, to original and inherited differences in bodily organization, or are they, rather, to be attributed to the customs, habits, and modes of life of the two classes of people?*

Some years ago, Henry I. Bowditch, of Boston, put on foot an extended system of inquiry in regard to ascertaining the causes or antecedents of consumption in the State of Massachusetts. In answer to some of the questions of the circular, Rabbi Dr. Guinzburg, of Boston, answered as follows, under date of October 29, 1872:

1. The number of Jews living in Boston is about 5000.
2. There certainly have not died of consumption, during the last five years, more than eight or ten Jews in the various congregations.

To this Dr. Bowditch adds, as follows:

> *If Dr. Guinzburg's data be correct, they show a very great immunity from consumption on the part of the Jews, compared with the citizens generally, as will be seen by the following comparison between these numbers and those procured from the Registration Reports, published by the State. In the report published in 1869, page 64, we find that for the five years preceding 1869 the annual average of deaths by consumption was 338 for every 100,000 living. These data from Dr. Guinzburg and the State Report give the following table:*
> *Proportion of Deaths to 100,000 of Living.*
> *All religions, 338*
> *Jews, 40*

These statements from Dr. Guinzburg are confirmed by the following letter from Dr. A. Haskins, of this city. Dr. Haskins is connected with one of the Jewish benevolent associations for the benefit of the sick. I sent to him similar questions and make the following extracts from his reply:

> *I am generally employed in about sixty families (Jewish). I have had these families under my care for two and a half years. During this time I have seen but one case of consumption. I have averaged among these sixty families about two visits daily. In my*

other Jewish practice, which is not inconsiderable, I have in this time (two and a half years) seen two cases of consumption.... I am sorry I have no statistics whereby I could compare the two peoples, viz., Jews and Christians. I can, therefore, give you only my impressions. I should say that I find consumption less frequent among the Jews than among Christians. This would be my own impression without any data to fortify it.

Dr. Waterman also sustains the same idea. The following extract will give some idea of his opportunities for observation and the sources of his deductions:

BOSTON, November 2, 1872. Dear Sir— ... First, I have attended four charitable associations; number about forty, fifty, sixty, and one hundred families. At present I only attend one, containing one hundred families, and on which I average a fraction over one visit a day. I have, besides, many private families among the Jews. I have attended but few cases of consumption, and I think the disease is not so relevant as among Christians.

The same report of Dr. Bowditch quotes from Stallard's *London Pauperism Amongst Jews and Christians*, as saying that there is no hereditary syphilis, and scarcely any scrofula to augment the mortality in the

Jewish families.

In relation to the liability of the Hebrew race to phthisis, Richardson has the following at page 22 of his *Diseases of Modern Life*:

> *The special inroads on vitality made on other races by disease are not easily determined, because of the difficulties arising from temporary admixture of race. I tried once to elicit some facts from a large experience of a particular disease, phthisis pulmonalis, and, as the results of this attempt may be useful, I put them briefly on record.*
>
> *At a public institution at which large numbers of persons afflicted with chest diseases applied for medical assistance, and at which I was for many years one of the physicians, I made notes during a short portion of the time of the connection that existed between race and the particular disease I have instanced—phthisis pulmonalis, or pulmonary consumption. The number of persons observed under the disease was three hundred, and no person was put on the record who was not suffering from a malady pure and simple; I mean without complication with any other malady. They who were thus studied were of four classes: (a) those who were by race distinctly Saxon; (b) those who were of mixed race, or whose race could not be determined; (c) those who were distinctly*

Celtic; (d) those who were distinctly Jewish. The results were, that of the three hundred patients, one hundred and thirty-three, 44.33 per cent., were Saxon; one hundred and eighteen, 39.33 per cent., were of mixed or undetermined race; thirty-one, 10.33 per cent., were Celtic; and eighteen, 6 per cent., were Jewish.

Although Dr. Richardson admits it would be unfair to accept the above figures as a basis for general application, he argues that they are, on the average, sufficiently suggestive, as among the Saxons it was noticed that there were more cases in whom the disease was hereditary, while among the others it was generally acquired.

In going over the subject of this question in regard to phthisis, we must admit that, although the Jew in his own home, synagogue, or in his social reunions, is not exposed to tubercular emanations, and that he has less chance of contracting the disease from tuberculous meats, he is, after all, a theatre-goer; a pretty constant inhabitant of the sleeping-car and hotel, as a commercial traveler and general merchant; and that, on the whole, he eats the same food, breathes the air and dust of the same streets, and drinks the same milk and water as the Christian, and, as observed by Dr. Billings, cooking destroys the bacillus in meats.

So that the comparative exposure in this country—where the practice is not as prevalent as in Germany of eating raw minced-meat sandwiches—existing between the Jew and the Christian to tubercular infection from meat are about equal. The records of the Jewish Hospital of New York gives, out of 28,750 persons admitted, only 44.17 per 1000 of its admissions as being due to consumption; while those of the Roosevelt Hospital, out of 25,583 admissions, gives a per 1000 of 67.93.

From what is known of the relation of syphilis to consumption, not only as affecting the primary individual, but the subsequent generations of the same, and the known greater exemption of the Jew to syphilitic infection, owing to the protecting influence of circumcision, it is safe to assert that therein is to be found one of the main reasons of the exemption of that race to consumption. If we but look at the geographical distribution of phthisis and the history of its progress, we shall find that it has had syphilis as its *avant courrier* on more than one occasion.

Lancereaux, in his *Distribution of Pulmonary Phthisis*, points to the fact that where consumption has made its greatest ravages, and where it has nearly depopulated one of the great divisions of the globe— namely, the groups of islands in the Pacific Ocean— the disease had no existence at the beginning of the present century.

Syphilis, scrofula, and a quick, galloping consumption have, since the last ninety years, taken off the greater part of the population. The same course of transition from the best of physical conditions to racial deterioration and extinction from the same relative condition of causes—syphilis, scrofula, and phthisis—has been observed among the open-air dwellers of the New Mexican Plains, in the mountains of Arizona, and on the arid wastes of the Colorado

Desert, where the appearance of consumption cannot be attributed to housing or incipient civilization, as it is attributed to housing among the Chippeways, Sioux, or Mandans in the regions that formerly formed the Northwest Territory.

The question is very plainly answered as to how consumption was introduced or whence it sprung that has so ravaged the Oceanic Islands. The sailors who first visited those islands were not, as a rule, a batch of consumptive tourists on a voyage in search of health or recreation; but we can well understand that the proverbially improvident mariner has not always had his health looked after by an Anson or a Cook, and that many a festive tar who induced the unsophisticated Indian maid to join him in worship at the shrine of Venus Porcina carried in the innermost recesses of the folds of his pendulous and sea-beaten prepuce the remnants of former Bacchanalian festivities performed in the questionable temples of Venus and Bacchus in Portsmouth or London.

Consumption, as such, was neither imported nor propagated by Europeans into those islands, its original entry being in the shape of syphilis. Had it been the ancient mariners of old Phoenicia in the days of its circumcision, or the circumcised marines of the ancient Atlantean fleets from the sunken continent of Plato, instead of the uncircumcised sailors of modern England, that first and since visited those islands, it is safe to say that consumption would not now exist there.

From this, it may be well to inquire what would be the relation between the Jewish race and consumption; were circumcision among them to be done away with, would it not be greatly on the increase?

The weight of testimony is evidently convincing that the Jew has a greater longevity and stronger resistance to disease, as well as a less liability to physical ills, than other races; that all these exemptions or benefits are not altogether due to social customs is evident; how much circumcision may have to do in inducing these favorable conditions can be better appreciated by a consideration of how circumcision affects those of other races, and more particularly how its performance works changes in the individual in his general health and condition, and in doing away with many physical ailments that the individual was previously subjected to.

So that the Jew cannot be said to be a loser by his observance of this rite, and he and his race have been well repaid for all the sufferings and persecutions that its observance has subjected them to.

As observed by John Bell,

> *The preservation of health and the attainment of long life are objects of desire to every man, no matter in what age or country his lot is cast, nor by what arbitrary tenure he holds his life. They are the wish of the master and the slave, of the illiterate and the learned, of the timid Hindoo and the warlike Arab, of the natives of New Zealand not less than of the inhabitants of New England—an indispensable condition for the greatest and longest enjoyment of the senses and propensities; for the widest range and*

exercise of intellect and gratification of the sentiments, whether these be lofty or ignoble, health, in any special degree, has ever been a fit subject of contemplation and instruction by the philosopher and legislator. Their advice and edicts on the means of preserving it have frequently been enforced as a part of religious duty, and, at all times, civilization, even in its elementary forms, has been marked by laws on this head. With the numerous and minute hygienic enactments of the great Jewish lawgiver for the guidance of the people of Israel we are all familiar. Prompted, we may suppose, in part by the example of Moses, and also by considerations growing out of the nature of the climate in which he lived, Mohammed incorporated with the mingled reveries, ethics, and blasphemies, which composed his Koran, dietetic rules and observances of regimen that are to this day implicitly obeyed by his zealous followers.[71]

If circumcision is not a factor in the difference that exists between the Jewish race and other races, if it goes for nothing as an exemptor of disease and the promoter of longevity, then there must exist some other factor or cause that induces these conditions.

What this factor is, the legislator, the sociologist, and the physician should make it their business to

---

[71] *On Regimen and Longevity*, John Bell, M.D. Page 13.

find out.

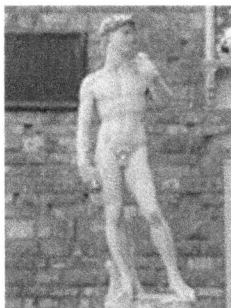

CHAPTER XV—PREDISPOSITION TO AND EXEMPTION AND IMMUNITY FROM DISEASE

The peculiar differences that exist between different animals in regard to their susceptibility to the action of drugs is even more remarkable than the differences that exist in their susceptibility to certain forms of disease.

We can understand and appreciate what Koch tells us in regard to the different susceptibilities exhibited by the house-mice and the field-mice to the anthrax bacillus, or why a nursing child should offer different results, when exposed to the diphtheria bacillus or the contagious poison of any of the exanthemata, from those witnessed in the meat or promiscuously dieted child.

We can also appreciate that different individuals have different susceptibilities to disease, as well as we understand that the same degree is not always in an unvarying point of resistance or susceptibility in the same individual. The investigation and study of these conditions teach us, however, that there is a cause, or that there are causes that induce and modify this susceptibility. But there are conditions that are as yet beyond our comprehension. Take, for instance, two animals, both vertebrates, mammals, and dwelling together, eating the same food, and even having a mutual understanding or sympathy of mind and affections, having a like circulation, a like brain and nervous system, it would naturally be supposed that these two would exhibit a like susceptibility to the actions of narcotic poisons; but when we are told that one dog has taken 21 grains of atropia with impunity we are staggered.

Atropia may not affect rabbits (as it does not), but the rabbit does not approach man in the same close relationship as the dog. Richardson administered to a healthy young cat 7 drachms of Battley's solution of opium, then 10 grains of morphia, and a little later 20 grains more of morphia without rendering the cat unconscious.

The same experimenter gave to a pigeon 21, 30, and 40, then 50 grains of powdered opium on succeeding days with no bad effect. S. Weir Mitchell gave to three pigeons, respectively, 272 drops of black drop, 21 grains of powdered opium, and 3 grains of morphia without any effect.[72]

On the other hand, horses show a like susceptibility to man to the action of drugs. In the island of Ceylon, a sloth can take 10 grains of strychnia with safety—chickens presenting a like

---

[72] *British and Foreign Medico-Chirurgical Review*, vol. xliii, page 539.

immunity to the poisonous effects of this alkaloid. While the dog offers such a contrast to the action of drugs as compared to man, he is as subject to goitre, and they have been seen in a true state of cretinism.[73]

An Apache, or Colorado Indian, will prefer a dessert of decomposed gophers to one composed of the best canned peaches or Bartlett pears; he will devour the mass without any resulting evil, while a German— after many generations of training on all forms of sausages in every degree of age and ripeness, and on every form of cheese, from the refreshing cottage cheese from curdled milk and the delicious cream cheese, down through to all and every grade as far as Limburgher, or maggoty, common cheese—has not, in every case overcome the tendency of the civilized intestine and constitution to the action of sausage poison, something that has no effect on the ordinary Indian, or on the uncivilized dweller north of the arctic circle.

Even the house-dog, that faithful companion of man, in many cases living on exactly the same fare as his master, is insensible to the action of this poison. An Indian will gorge and gormandize, after a prolonged fast, on such quantities and qualities of food that, if the ordinary white man were to indulge in a like feast, he would be in imminent danger of literal rupture or explosion, or liable to end in sudden apoplectic seizures, or, in case of a too healthy and active digestion, liable, owing to a lack of a correspondingly active condition of the excretory organs, to go off in uræmic coma.

---

[73] *Ibid.*, vol. xlii, page 17.

Peter Charles Remondino

This sporadic and fitful feasting has no perceptible effect on the Indian, who either simply works it off in exercise, or sleeps it off in a long and prolonged period of sleep, during which his lungs work with the deep and steady pull and persistence that a tug-boat exhibits when towing in a large ship against the tide and a head wind—working in and out more air in one respiration than the ordinary white man will in a dozen.

All these different conditions are more or less plain to us and as easy of explanation—just as plain as to how and why some birds eat gravel to improve their digestion. In the cases of different susceptibility to the action of strychnia or of narcotics, the explanation must of necessity, for the present, be more or less speculative. But how are we to account, even in the way of speculation, for the peculiar immunity, lack of predisposition and hereditary tendencies to disease exhibited by the Hebrew, who, since the history of the world, has been a civilized and rational being—even for decades of centuries before the civilization of Europe?

Living under the same forms of government, climate, and shelter, practically using the same varieties of food and drink, he exhibits an entirely different vitality and resistance to disease, decay, and death—being, in fact, a puzzle to the demographic student. The only really marked difference that exists between this race and the others lies in the fact that the Hebrew is circumcised, other differences not being sufficiently constant to be accounted as factors.

Circumcision is, in the opinion of the writer, the real cause of the differences in longevity and faculty for the enjoyment of life that the Hebrew enjoys in contrast to his Christian brother. Christian and uncircumcised races may individually, or in classes, develop some peculiar immunity or exemption, as, for instance, the tolerance to arsenic exhibited by some German mountaineers, or the peculiar safety enjoyed by the butcher class from attacks of continued fever;[74][74] but these exemptions are purchased at the expense of the future, the effects of arsenic, long continued, finally having its morbid effects, and the very plethora which is the bulwark of resistance in the butcher, this plethora being in the end a treacherous foe, diseases result from it which make a sudden ending to this class when it is least expected.

For an all around long-liver the Hebrew holds a pre-eminence, and, as the factor in this pre-eminence, circumcision has no counter-claimant.

Circumcision is like a substantial and well-secured life-annuity; every year of life you draw the benefit, and it has not any drawbacks or after-claps. Parents cannot make a better paying investment for their little boys, as it insures them better health, greater capacity for labor, longer life, less nervousness, sickness, loss of time, and less doctor-bills, as well as it increases their chances for an euthanasian death.

---

[74] In *Influence of the Trades on Health*, Thakrah mentions the peculiar exemption enjoyed in this regard by the butcher class. He quotes Tweedie in saying that he never saw a butcher admitted to the fever hospital.

Peter Charles Remondino

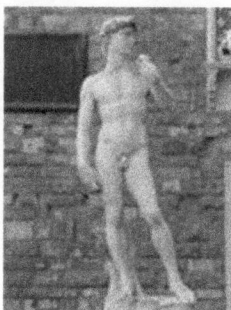

CHAPTER XVI—THE PREPUCE, SYPHILIS, AND PHTHISIS

It is not alone the tight-constricted, glans-deforming, onanism-producing, cancer-generating prepuce that is the particular variety of prepuce that is at the bottom of the ills and ailments, local or constitutional, that may affect man through its presence.

The loose, pendulous prepuce, or even the prepuce in the evolutionary stage of disappearance, that only loosely covers one-half of the glans, is as dangerous as his long and constricted counterpart. If we look over the world's history, since in the latter years of the fifteenth century syphilis came down like a plague, walking with democratic tread through all walks and stations in life, laying out alike royalty or the vagrant, the curled-haired and slashed-doubleted knight, or the tonsured monk, we must conclude that syphilis has caused more families to become extinct than any ordinary plague, black death, or cholera epidemic.

Without wishing to enter into a history of syphilis, it is not outside of the province of this book to allude to its frequency and spread.

Syphilis is not restricted to classes by any means; it is not those of the lower class alone who are its victims. Dr. Fr. J. Behrend, in his work, *Die Prostitution in Berlin*, observes that abolition of the brothels in that city in 1845, '46, '47 and '48, trebled the number of cases of syphilis treated at the Der Charité; in the year 1848 the cases of syphilis treated at that hospital numbered over 1800.

It was also remarked during this period of legally-enforced virtue, that, as inconsistently as it might appear, the disease invaded the best of families. From Dr. Neumann, in his brochure entitled *Die Berliner Syphilisfrage*, published in 1852, we learn that, in the Trades and Mechanics' Benevolent Union of Berlin, in 1849, 13.51 percent of the sick were so from syphilis.

In the thirteenth volume of the *British and Foreign Medico-Chirurgical Review*, we find, in a review of the control of prostitution, an estimate in regard to the syphilization of a nation. The estimates are made on the most conservative figures, as, in the desire of the reviewer not to overestimate, he starts by figuring out the actual number of prostitutes in England, Wales, and Scotland to be only 50,000, when they were estimated, by those who had carefully studied the subject, as being more than double that number; the conservative estimate is, however, suitable for our purpose; so that we cannot be accused of overestimating the results.

The portion of the review to which we wish to call attention is as follows:

Though the result of the evidence contained

in the first report of the commissioners on the constabulary force of England and Wales was that at that time about 2 percent of the prostitutes of London were suffering under some form of venereal disease, yet we will descend even lower, and presume that of one hundred healthy prostitutes, taken promiscuously from England and Scotland, if each submits to one indiscriminate sexual act in twenty-four hours, not more than one would become infected with syphilis, an estimate which is without doubt far too low; yet, if admitted to be correct, the necessary consequence will be, that of the fifty thousand prostitutes five hundred are diseased within the aforesaid twenty-four hours.

If we next admit that a fifth of these five hundred diseased women are admitted to hospital on the day on which the disease appears, it follows that there are every day on the streets four hundred diseased women. Let it be supposed that the power of these four hundred to infect be limited to twelve days, and that of every six persons who, at the rate of one each night, have connection with these women, five become infected, it will follow that there will be four thousand men infected every night, and consequently one million four hundred and sixty thousand in the year. Further, as there are every night four hundred women diseased by these men, one hundred and eighty-two thousand five hundred public prostitutes will be syphilized during the year; hence, one million six hundred and fifty-two thousand five hundred cases of syphilis in both sexes occur every twelve months.

If, then, the entire population had intercourse with prostitutes in an equal ratio, the gross population of Great Britain, of all ages and sexes, would, during eighteen years, have been affected with primary syphilis. Be it remembered, we do not assert that more than a million and a half of persons are attacked every year, but that that number of cases occurs annually in England, Wales, and Scotland, though the same individual may be attacked more than once. Although it is evident that all the estimates used for these calculations are (we know no other word that expresses it) ridiculously low, yet we find that more than a million and a half of cases of syphilis occur every year—an amount which is probably not half the actual number. How enormous, then, must be the number of children born with secondary disease! How immense the mortality among them! How vast an amount of public and private money expended on the cure of this disease!

The same reviewer (P. S. Holland), in another article on the *Control of Prostitution*, observes that among the

British troops syphilis is one of the most frequent of diseases, about one hundred and eighty cases occurring annually among every one thousand soldiers.

The effect of syphilis in depopulating the islands of the Pacific has been pointed out in a former chapter; the nature and origin of the disease that takes them off is unmistakable. Scrofula and rapid phthisis are taking off the inhabitants at a rate that, in those islands most affected, the native population will soon become extinct.

According to Lancereaux, in the Marquesas group the women do not live beyond the age of thirty to thirty-five years, three or four months being the duration of the disease. Ellis, in his *Polynesian Researches*, published in 1836, remarks that at that date the disease, as above described, had but recently appeared. In the nineteenth volume of the *Archives de Médecine Navale*, Rey mentions that at the Easter Island pulmonary phthisis is the dominant affection with the adults, and that scrofula is very prevalent with the children.[75]

The effect of syphilization in inducing a scrofulous taint and the appearance of a rapidly-marching consumption among savage races has been well observed among the Indians in the southwestern parts of the United States, where the appearance of these fatal diseases can easily be traced to that as a cause.

There is something peculiar about the Anglo-Saxon race that is fatal to the Indian; wherever they come in contact, the savage race begins physically and morally to crumble; the habits of the Anglo-Saxon in the

---

[75] *Distribution de la Phthisie Pulmonaire*, Lancereaux.

matter of intemperance and his lust soon end the poor Indian; while, on the other hand, the Latin races mix with them without any physical detriment to the Indian.

In what was formerly the Northwest Territory the French and Indian intermarried, and syphilis did not begin to tell on the Indian until the Americans settled the country. From these observations it is very evident that in the Polynesian Archipelago syphilis must have been the precursor of the phthisis and scrofula, as we know it to have been that which induced those diseases among the Indians of the Mississippi or Missouri Valleys, or of the Colorado and Mojave Deserts, or in the mountains and valleys of Arizona.

On the other hand, circumcised races, whose women have not carried a syphilitic taint into the race, are as a class free from any syphilitic taint. Neither their teeth, physiognomy, skin, nor general condition denote any syphilitic inheritance. This is true of the Jewish descendants of Abraham, who have more strictly adhered to the non-intercourse or marriage with other races, and whose women have abstained from vice; the Arabian descendants of Ishmael have, in a great measure, also retained their marked family individuality, except it be a few tribes, who, by contact with the soldiery of European nations, have had their women corrupted and syphilis introduced into the tribe through this channel.

Richardson, in his *Preventive Medicine*, observing on the effects of syphilis in inducing deterioration of the organs of circulation and their degenerative changes, says that, in his opinion, syphilis is the progenitor of various diseases, and that those who give this opinion the greatest range are, unfortunately, nearest the truth. The breathing organs, he remarks, are distinctly susceptible to injury from this hereditary cause.

In 1854, at the Metropolitan Free Hospital, situated in the Jews' quarter in London, Hutchinson observed that the proportion of Jews to Christians among the out-patients was as one to three; at the same time the proportion of cases of syphilis in the former to the latter was one to fifteen. Now, this result was not due to any extra morality on the part of the Jews, as fully one-half of the gonorrhoea cases occurred among those of that faith. J. Royes Bell also observes the less syphilization among circumcised races.[76]

The absence of the prepuce and the non-absorbing character of the skin of the glans penis, made so by constant exposure, with the necessary and unavoidably less tendency that these conditions give to favor syphilitic inoculation, are not evidently without their resulting good effects.

Now and then syphilitic primary sores are found on the glans, or even in the urethra or on the outside skin of the penis, or outer parts of the prepuce; but the majority are, as a rule, situated either back of the corona or on the reflected inner fold of the prepuce immediately adjoining the corona, or they may be in the loose folds in the neighborhood of the frenum, the retention of the virus seemingly being assisted by the topographical condition and relation of the parts, and its absorption facilitated by the thinness of the

---

[76] *Int. Enc. Surgery*, Ashhurst.

mucous membrane, as well as by the active circulation and moisture and heat of the parts.

It must be evident that but for these favoring conditions the inoculation or infection would and could not be either as sure or as frequent. Any protecting mechanical aid that interferes with these favoring conditions grants an immunity to the individual, even when he is freely exposed; this protection has often been obtained by applying to the glans and penis a substantial coat of some tenacious oil like castor-oil, which was afterward gently washed off, first in a shower of tepid water and afterward in a tepid bath of warm water and borax.

Horner, formerly of the navy, in his interesting little work on *Naval Practice*, [77] relates that it was customary, in the older navy of the United States, to allow public women to come on board at some of the ports and to go down to the men between decks, the Department of the Navy being probably actuated by the same humane principle that used to induce some of the West Indian cannibals to lend their wives to their prisoners of war who were intended, in the shape of roast or *fricandeau*, to grace the festive board, as it was deemed inhuman by these philanthropists to deprive a man of his necessary sexual intercourse, even if they were soon to roast him and pick his bones.

They may, however, have been selfish in the matter, as by some authorities it is represented that this was done to improve the flavor of the prisoner, who was said to offer a more savory dish through this

---

[77] *Naval Practice*, Horner.

considerate treatment, the strong flavor that the semen gives to flesh being well eradicated by free fornication.

Whether it was through these motives of humanitarianism, or the feeling that an American tar was the equal of the British tar, whose praises and equality Sir Joseph Porter, K.C.B., writes a song about in *Pinafore*, who had as much right to contract a left-handed marriage as any Prince of Wales or any other prince or crowned head of Europe, the women were, nevertheless, allowed to go down between decks in preference to giving the men indiscriminate liberty on shore, the government further providing for their welfare by causing the assistant surgeon to examine the women at the gangway or hatchway, to see that they were not diseased.

Horner relates the ludicrous appearance presented by a near-sighted assistant at one of the hatchways while making this professional examination, surrounded by the sailors and marines, who were greatly-interested spectators. Had the government provided a pot of castor-oil wherein the tar could dip his penile organ, as bridge piles are dipped into a creasoting mixture, these humiliations to our professional brother could have been avoided.

In the conclusion to be reached, circumcision is not put forward as the only exempting element or preventive measure that deserves all the credit for the immunity that the Jews enjoy from syphilis, or to the absence of hereditary diseases that are secondary or due to the presence of that disease in the parents, as considerable credit is to be given to the well-known chastity of their females.

This chastity is, in a great measure, due to the inseparable conditions of their religion—moral and social fabrics which are welded into one. Their charity assumes the most practical form, so that it is not possible for one of their females to have to resort to a life of prostitution to save herself or her children from starvation, as, unfortunately, is too often the case in Christian communities, where religion is put on and off with Sunday clothes.

The temperance and sobriety, as well as the economy and industry of the father, are not without a good moral as well as a hereditary effect on the daughters, who are neither rendered brutal nor demoralized through the example and instigation of drunken fathers.

They have, therefore, a better average homelife, to which they cling and which protects them. The aid and benevolent associations of the Jews are among the most efficacious of charitable institutions, and no class gives more freely or generously for this purpose. The Home for Aged Hebrews in New York is an example of the character with which they dispense charity. We need not, therefore, be surprised to find, in statistics of illegitimacy by religious denominations taken in Prussia, that the Jewish women are three times as chaste as the Catholics and more than four times as chaste as the Evangelists.[78] The Jew has, therefore, two avenues of infection from syphilis cut off—the lesser liability due to his circumcision and the chastity of the women.

Richardson mentions the immunity of the Jewish

---

[78] *Cincinnati Lancet and Observer*, vol. xvi, 1873.

race from tubercular disease, and notices the well-known relation existing between a syphilitic taint and a phthisical tendency. The comparative statistics offered by the Mohammedans, Jews, and Christians in regard to deaths from consumption have already been mentioned in a former chapter, they being as four Christians to one Jew, while the Mohammedan, from his greater abstemiousness and temperance to assist him, shows a still lower percentage than the Jew.

There can be but little doubt that to this particular and well-marked less syphilization the Hebrew race owes much of its exemption from many other diseases and its greater resistance to ordinary ailments and epidemic diseases.

The relative less frequency of syphilis among all circumcised people is noticed by Dr. Bernheim, in his brochure *De la Circoncision,* he being the surgeon of the Israelitish Consistory of Paris. His utterances on this subject are worthy of attention, he having not only paid particular attention to this, but having had unusual opportunities for the basis of his opinions.

Dr. Bernheim looks upon coition as a frequent source of tubercular infection, and the sensitive and absorbing covering of the uncircumcised glans as a ready medium of transmission of the virus from one system to the other. He calls attention to the frequent granular condition of the uterine os, in confirmed cases of tuberculosis, as something that is too much overlooked. This view of the case, from Dr. Bernheim's stand-point, is worthy of greater consideration than it has generally received at the hands of the profession.

The great number of examples that have recently come to light in connection with the direct inoculability of tubercular consumption, both in the later works on phthisis and in the medical press, are not without interest or without a lesson.

The case recorded within the past year of a healthy chambermaid, who was immediately inoculated with tubercular matter with rapidly-following constitutional effects through a scratch on the hand, received from the sharp edge of a broken china cuspidor that a consumptive was using, is one of these cases that are to the point; so it is evident that the uncircumcised need not always wait for the degeneration of syphilis into syphilitic phthisis or syphilitic scrofula to become a consumptive, but it is within the greatest range of possibility and probability that he may become at once a consumptive through an excoriation or abrasion received during coition with a tubercular woman.

So many tubercular prostitutes ply their trade, or, to be more definite, so many prostitutes become tubercular, and in its different stages follow their occupation as the only means of keeping out of the poor-house, that man runs as much if not more risk, in consorting with the class, of contracting tuberculosis than that of contracting syphilis.

There is something about syphilis that is not generally noticed; we are all well acquainted with the dire results that usually follow syphilitic infection, its course through every stage of suffering and misery, its transmission and effects in tubercular meningitis or in syphilitic affections of the mesentery through heredity in children, and of the many horrible cases of destruction of tissue, in skin, mucous membrane, cartilage, or bone, with their attending mutilations and disfigurations; but there is no record of the great number of cases, and very few physicians of any extended practice but who can recall some such cases, where, after undoubted syphilitic infection, with the usual course of primary sores and secondary eruption, the patient has suddenly blossomed out into a state of robust health that his system was an entire stranger to before the infection.

The writer has, in the course of a long practice, seen a number of such results follow both the infection attended with a miliary eruption and that followed by the large small-pox-appearing eruption, both kinds being preceded by the primary sore; and these results have been observed in cases of both what are called the soft and multiple and the hard or Hunterial initial sore. Some of these cases rapidly gained in flesh, with an evident increase in the redness of their blood, increasing in vigor and strength with a very perceptibly less tendency to attacks from accidental or previously subject-to diseases.

The same result has been observed to follow an attack of small-pox with some individuals, and the writer well remembers a similar result following a very extraordinary event.

The subject was a man well known among his old comrades of the First Minnesota Infantry as "Duke," and to many of the older practitioners of Wabashaw County, of that State, as "Old Duke." In early life he was sickly and weakly, never having fully recovered from a malarial fever contracted in the Mexican war. Coming to Minnesota, he adopted the life of a raftsman, with all the irregularities that accompanied such a life.

On one occasion, after a protracted spree, feeling the need of stimulation and not having the wherewith to procure it, he secured a jar in which a snake and several other reptiles were preserved in spirits, and drank the fluid contents.

He was, some days afterward, taken violently ill with a high fever and racking pains, ending in an eruption of boils that covered him from head to foot; he made a slow and tedious recovery; but when recovered he seemed to have become imbued with a constitution resembling *lignum-vitæ*, for a more stubborn-twisted constitution never existed than that of "Old Duke." The power of resistance that this man developed was something wonderful.

Dr. C. P. Adams, of Hastings, Minnesota, and the St. Paul physicians who were connected with the regiment well remember, though, wiry, precise, and soldierly "Duke," who, even in the old Army of the Potomac, immersed up to his ears like the rest of the army in the mud and dirt of the encampment of Falmouth, above Fredericksburg, came out on general inspection as prim as if he had just stepped out of a bandbox, for which he received a medal for soldierly conduct and bearing.

These apparent digressions are not made either to be tedious or to weary the reader, nor without an object. They are made to show that, whereas syphilis is looked upon as such a deadly disease, and it may be said to be the sole cause of fear to the assiduous worshiper at the shrine of Venus Porcina, there is another still more fatal danger awaiting him, ambushed in the folds of the vaginal mucous membrane, or coming along silently out of the cervical canal—like the legions of Cyrus stealing along the dry bed of the Euphrates into ancient Babylon, to fall unawares on the feasting Nebuchadnezzar on that fatal night.

So, in like manner, the virus of tuberculosis, either extruding from a granular os or from its neighborhood, gradually moves down on the unsuspecting, uncircumcised, and easily inoculable-surfaced glans penis, to infect the system with a tubercular poison that has no such exceptions as those above noted, as at times are the followers of syphilis.

It is not alone the individual himself that may be the sufferer from this poison, but his progeny for several generations may have to suffer for the infection thus received, just as much as they would were that infection to have been syphilitic. As before remarked, this has heretofore not sufficiently occupied the consideration of the profession, and, as it cannot certainly be denied that such a source of tubercular infection is both possible and probable, the subject is entitled to more serious and deliberate consideration than that which has heretofore been paid to it.

Tuberculosis certainly has these two channels of entrance: either through direct infection or through an evolutionary process resulting from syphilis. The appearance and vital statistics offered by the French War Office in regard to the Algierine provinces, the report of the United States Census, the opinion of Dr. Billings deduced from the census reports, the opinions of Hutchinson, Richardson, Bernheim, and many other observers, as well as the personal but unrecorded observations of many practitioners, all tend to bear testimony to the remarkable difference that exists between circumcised and uncircumcised races in regard to the ravages of consumption.

Is circumcision a factor in this difference, or is it not? If it is, then circumcision should receive more attention than it has; if it is not, then we should not be idle in hunting up the cause of difference, for an ounce of prevention is certainly worth in this regard a whole pound of Koch's lymph as a curative agent.

Peter Charles Remondino

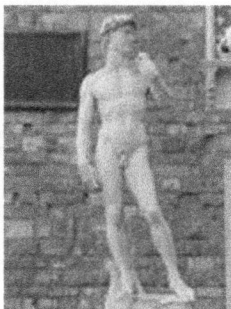

CHAPTER XVII—SOME REASONS FOR BEING CIRCUMCISED

The surgical and medical history of circumcision is intimately connected with the remotest ages, this being, in fact, the earliest surgical procedure of which we have any record. From the same records we obtain hints as to two conditions for which circumcision probably was suggested, either as a preventive or as a remedy.

Jahn, in speaking of the people by whom the early Hebrews were surrounded, mentions their idolatrous practices, and that their peculiar forms of Pagan worship were accompanied by indulgence in fornication, lascivious songs, and unnatural lust. Others of their neighbors worshiped the *hairy he-goat*, with which they also practiced all manner of abominations.

Sodomy, or pederasty, seemed a sort of religious ceremony with some of these heathen nations; from a religion it necessarily became a social practice; this, in connection with the phallic practices and worship, necessitated frequent exposure of the male member. The evil results, to say nothing of the disgusting and demoralizing tendency of these practices of the Pagan, were evidently well known to the Jews.

The contrast between the physique and health of the pastoral habits, out-of-door life and simple diet of the Jews, and the necessary opposite condition of health and physique due to luxury and to these practices among their neighbors, could not have escaped their attention. How much onanism had to do with the establishment of circumcision may well be conjectured.

Again, the other hint is in reference to procreation, as some stress is laid to the connection between the conception of Sarah and the circumcision of Abraham. Here we have suggestions of a preventive to onanism, and a cure to male impotence when due to preputial interference.[79]

Strange as it may seem, these two important results, due to circumcision, seem to have been lost sight of for some thousands of years, as even the able works of the physicians of the latter part of the last century have nothing to say connecting onanism and circumcision.

Neither the works of Tissot on male onanism nor

---

[79] It may well be a question of some interest whether the atrophy of the testicle in the aged may not at times be partly due to the compression exercised by the prepuce on the glans through reflex action, and whether at times the virility that is departing cannot be restored by circumcision in such cases. I have seen such results, being guided to the idea by the Biblical relation in the case of Abraham.

the pioneer work of Bienville on nymphomania speak of the presence of the prepuce in the male, or of the nymphar or clitorian prepuce in the female, as being causative of, or their removal curative of, either masturbation, satyriasis, or nymphomania; moral, hygienic, and internal medication being by both these authors considered to be all that our science could offer or do to alleviate or cure this unfortunate class.

It is only of late years that circumcision, in its true relations to onanism, has received full consideration. In regard to its being a cure of impotence, its recognition has been of longer duration.

It is related by Leonard, in his *Memoires*—who, in his capacity of hair-dresser in ordinary to her Majesty, the unfortunate Marie-Antoinette, had ample opportunity for picking up all the domestic small talk of the royal family and their affairs—that Louis XVI, in addition to all his troubles and the indignities which he suffered, besides finally being beheaded, was afflicted with a congenital phimosis which prevented the flow of semen from properly discharging itself.

It appears that his Majesty was no little annoyed at not being able to procure an heir to his throne. His royal sister-in-law, the Countess d'Artois, had given birth to a prince, the Duke of Angouleme, who was the heir presumptive to the throne in case of the non-issue from Louis; another sister-in-law had been brought to bed with a royal princess, and here was the king himself without any prospective possibility of any heir.

Like all kings, he was more or less unreasonable; so he blamed his first surgeon in ordinary for all these short-comings—as if it were the duty of these court surgeons, among their many other tribulations, to furnish heirs to thrones. The surgeon finally informed his Majesty that if he wished to become a father it would be necessary for him to submit to the slight operation that was the subject of the church festival of the first day of January, namely, the Feast of the Circumcision.

His most Christian Majesty entered a protest to this acknowledgment that there was anything in Judaism worth imitating. The surgeon insisted that the operation celebrated on the first of January would put him in a way to have the much-desired heir. The king finally waived all objections from any religious scruples, but could not be brought to look at the prospective operation with any sentiments of agreeable expectation.

The king finally became good-natured, and a touch of that plebeian jollity which at times made him quite agreeable spread over his features as he imagined the ludicrousness of the spectacle that would be presented by a king of France in the hands of these handlers of the scalpel, treating him like an African savage.

He took some days to consider the matter. On the next day he informed M. Louis, his first surgeon in ordinary, that he had decided on submitting to the operation, and the day and hour were fixed. The royal circumcision, however, never took place, as it is most likely that in the privacy of his chamber his Majesty worked, like many a plebeian or man of low degree had done before him and has done since, to bring a refractory prepuce to terms.

The king was somewhat of a mechanic, as his skill as a locksmith has passed into history; so that it is not unlikely that, with what little information he had on the subject, he managed to sufficiently dilate, by scarification and stretching, the preputial opening, as from the year 1778 the queen had three children.

Cases of attempted self-circumcision are not rarities, as people have some inexplicable idea that a self-inflicted cut is not as painful as one that is done by others. The writer well remembers being called to assist one of these domestic surgeons who had undertaken to circumcise himself with his wife's great scissors.

The man had a very long but thin and narrow prepuce that had always been an annoyance to him. The writer had circumcised two of his children for the same malformation, and the father, seeing the benefit to these two, determined to share in the general benefit; but at the same time he arranged to do it all by himself, and give the family and the surgeon a sample of his courage and a simultaneous surprise party.

Securing the scissors, he wended his way unperceived into the recesses of his wood-shed. The mental and physical anguish the poor man underwent, and what soliloquies he must have addressed to the rafters of the wood-shed while making up his mind and screwing up his physical courage for the last fell act with the scissors, can hardly be described, as, in all probability, they were of the most rambling and inconsistent order.

At any rate, he must have reached a climax in time and grasped the fated prepuce with a revengeful glee, and, with all his powers concentrated in his good right hand, he must have closed the remorseless blades of the scissors on the unlucky prepuce. When the surgeon arrived at the scene of carnage, he was directed to the wood-shed, on the outskirts of which hovered the family, frantic with fear and apprehension; within, in the darkest corner, with wildly dilated eyes, and performing a fantastic *pas seul*, was a man with a huge pair of scissors dangling between his legs, warning all hands as they valued his life not to approach or lay a hand on him.

He had shut the scissors down so that it clinched the thin prepuce, and there his courage and determination had forsaken him; he lost his presence of mind, and was not even able to take off the scissors; he had simply given one wild, blood-curdling yell—like the last winding notes from Roland's horn at Roncevalles—that had brought his family to the wood-shed-door, and they had then sent for a surgeon.

New terrors here awaited the unlucky victim for self-circumcision. He dreaded lest the surgeon should accidentally have it enter his mind to finish the operation with the scissors, and in that case he would be helpless, as the surgeon would, undoubtedly, have a sure and tender hold of it.

After executing a number of *pas à deux* on the Magilton step, while the surgeon endeavored to reassure him and gain his confidence, promising to remove the scissors without inflicting any further harm, he was finally allowed to approach, and, while the patient assumed a Taglioni attitude on one foot, the other leg being extended at right angles with the body and his hands clawing the air, the scissors was removed. The patient, through the aid of lead lotions and a week's rest, made a good recovery with a whole prepuce, chagrined at his failure, but happy to have escaped immediate pain.[80]

There is not much doubt but that the operation could have been suggested by its, at times, spontaneous performance, a case of which, by Cullerier, and some other additional cases have been mentioned in a former chapter. Cases occur at times, also, wherein the person having a previously normal and uninterfering prepuce has, through either herpetic inflammations or through impure connection, spurious gonorrhoea, or the use of some venereal-disease preventing-wash after connection, produced some irritation resulting in the abnormal thickening of

---

[80] This patient subsequently died of a uræmic complication following on an attack of fever. The man was in his prime, and had been of most exemplary habits. The fever that he had was, I had every reason to believe, directly due to the results of imperfect blood depuration incident on the irritability of his kidneys, which, retroactively, again allowed the uræmic condition to assume that dangerous degree that suddenly and very unexpectedly to his friends and family ushered the patient into eternity. This man had only been merely inconvenienced by his prepuce up to the time that it caused his death. It is interesting to observe what little trifles bring about the end of some men. The unlucky habit of putting the royal countenance on paper brought Louis XVI to a sudden halt at Varennes, and his head to the scaffold. The lucky meeting of the *aides* of Bonaparte and Desaix between Novi and Marengo gave to France its empire and to Europe the enlightenment that was diffused by that event. If such trifles affect individuals and nations, we must not be astonished that the little useless prepuce should be endowed with the mischief-working power of the historical old cow and kerosene lamp that reduced Chicago to ashes.

the inner fold, or an interstitial deposit at the junction of the skin and mucous membrane, with consequent constriction, this deposit finally forming a hard, inelastic ring, which prevented a free exposure of the glans and interfered in sexual connection.

In such cases—like in stricture of the meatus—any mechanical interference short of cutting with a knife only aggravates the existing difficulty, and it is not uncommon to have such cases apply for assistance after they have in vain tried to dilate the constricting preputial orifice.

In the early writings of the Greeks, it is mentioned that among the Egyptians circumcision exempted them from a certain form of disease that affected the penis. Philon mentions particularly the immunity that the operation conferred against a species of affection which Michel Levy asserts to have been a gangrenous disease. So that, outside of any religious significance, there is no doubt that, in individual cases, circumcision has more than once been suggested, although it cannot be said that such individual cases would ever, or could, lead to its becoming a national or racial, much less a sectarian, rite.

Peter Charles Remondino

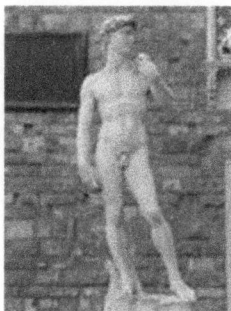

CHAPTER XVIII—THE PREPUCE AS AN OUTLAW, AND ITS EFFECTS ON THE GLANS

Ricord has well termed this appendage to civilized man *a useless bit of flesh.* Times were, however, when—man living in a wild state, and when in imitation of some of our near relatives with tails and hairy bodies; when he still found locomotion on all-fours handier than on his two feet; when in pursuit of either the juicy grasshopper or other small game, or of the female of his own species to gratify his lust, or in the frantic rush to escape the clutches, fangs, or claws of a pursuing enemy, he was obliged to fly and leap over thorny briars and bramble-bushes or hornets' nests, or plunge through swamps alive with blood-sucking insects and leeches—Ricord's definition would certainly have been inapplicable.

In those days, but for the protecting double fold of the preputial envelope that protected it from the thorns and cutting grasses, the coarse bark of trees, or the stings and bites of insects, the glans penis of primitive man would have often looked like the head of the proverbially duel-disfigured German university student, or the Bacchus-worshiping nose of a jolly British Boniface. So that in those days, unless primitive man was intended to have an organ that resembled a battle-scarred Roman legionary, a prepuce was an absolute necessity.

With improvement in man's condition and his gradual evolution into a higher sphere, the assumption of the erect posture, and the great stride in civilization that originated the invention of the manufacture of the perineal band, which not only protected the glans in its thorny passage through life, but also acted like a protecting ægis to the scrotum and its contents, the prepuce became a superfluity; not only a superfluity, but, now that its natural office had been replaced by the perineal cloth, it actually began to be a nuisance, as its former free contact with the air had retained it in a state of vigorous and disease-resisting health which was now fast departing.

As Montesquieu observes, in the causes that led to the decline and fall of the Roman Empire, those seasons of trials, tribulations, and struggle for existence are those of health and progress and healthy life, and the periods of luxury and idleness are those of degeneracy and decay. So with the prepuce, the luxury and idleness, voluptuousness and consequent feasting incident to its being supplanted in its original functions by the perineal cloth, which left it thenceforth unemployed, led it in the pathway of disease and death.

This first innovation in civilization was to the prepuce the beginning of its decay and fall. Like Belshazzar in his great banquet-hall in ancient

Babylon, the prepuce might have read the hand-writing on the wall, *Mene, Mene, Tekel, Upharsin,* and foreseen the gory end that awaited it. Like to other human affairs, however, even in his fallen estate a kind word can be said for the prepuce. Puzey, of Liverpool, has found it of extreme value, and even unequaled by any other part of the body, for furnishing skin-grafts,[81] these grafts showing a vitality that is simply phenomenal, considering the laxity of its tissues and its seemingly adipose character.

There is no doubt, however, that for skin-transplanting there is nothing superior to the plants offered by the prepuce of a boy, and where any large surface is to be covered this should undoubtedly be chosen, as offering the greatest and quickest success and the least chances of failure. This is really the only disadvantage that can be charged against circumcision, as in a strictly circumcised community they would be debarred from this great advantage.

An uncircumcised individual could be procured, however, to supply the deficiency. It is related that in the latter part of 1890, a Knight Templar, in Cincinnati, required a great supply of grafts or skin-plants to cover a largely-denuded surface, and that the whole of his Commandery chivalrously and generously supplied the needed skin-plants in a body. A few healthy prepuces would have been more efficacious.

---

[81] In the London *Lancet* for 1885 there is a very interesting communication at page 46 on this subject. There is no doubt but that the prepuce offers the best skin-grafting material.

In advising the use of the prepuce for these purposes it must not be overlooked that in case of a white man it would not do to use skin of any other color besides his own. We have no data to base any assertion as to the relative action of skin-grafts taken from Mongolians or Indians, but we have very reliable data in relation to the proliferating action of those of the negro,[82] which induces a growth of epidermis of its own kind; so that preputial grafts from the negro, combining the extra vitality and proliferation of the preputial tissue with the strong animal vitality of the negro, if applied to a white man, might not produce the most desirable cosmetic effects, especially if on one side of the countenance.

But, taken as a whole, when considered in its relation to onanism, nocturnal enuresis, preputial

---

[82] In the seventeenth volume (third series) of *Guy's Hospital Reports* there is a most interesting report at page 243 of a case of skin-grafting that was performed by Thomas Bryant. The case was an extensive ulcer resulting from an injury. Bryant took some skin-grafts from the man's arm and some from a colored man in an adjoining bed. The account gives the daily report as taken from the note-book of Mr. Clarke, and is accompanied by a colored plate to illustrate the subject; the proliferation of the black skin is astonishing. In closing the report Mr. Clarke says: "But in the figures depicted the amount of increase in the black patches will be well seen. In ten weeks the four or five pieces of black skin, which together were not larger than a grain of barley, had grown twentyfold, and in an another month the black patch was more than one inch long by half an inch broad, the black centres of cutification having clearly grown very rapidly by the proliferation of their own black cells."

calculus, syphilis, cancer, and a lot of nervous and other ailments, or induced abnormal physical conditions, we can really conclude that the days of the prepuce are past and gone, that it has outlived its usefulness, and that those whom a religious or civil ordinance or custom happily makes them rid of it are people to be greatly envied. As Sancho Panza remarked, "God bless the man who invented sleep," so we may well join in blessing the inventor of circumcision, as an event that has saved some parts of the human family from much ill and suffering.

Phimosis is an ancient attendant on our inheritance of the prepuce, we being, in fact, born with it; this is the rule. There are, however, exceptions to this rule, which, singularly enough, are found to be hereditary. The writer has met with a number of such instances, and they have always been found to have been family traits. Within the past year, after attending a confinement, his attention was called to the child by the nurse, who thought that the child was deformed; the nurse, singularly enough, never having seen a natural-looking glans penis in all her life, was astonished at the size and appearance of the member.

On examination, the organ showed a complete absence of prepuce. On inquiry, the father and another son, born more than twenty years previously— this comprising every male member of the family— were found to have been thus born, with the glans fully exposed. The family is now residing in San Diego, and is naturally one of more than superior physical health and intelligence.

I saw another family similarly affected in the north of France, and of individual cases, without knowing the history of the rest of the family, I have seen a large number. As the prepuce can be observed in every stage of disappearance among mixed races, it would seem that in time it would disappear altogether. Its effectual absence in so many cases evidently belongs to some evolutionary process, and shows beyond question that nature does not insist on its presence either as a necessity or as an ornament.

The word or term *phimosis* is derived from two Greek roots, signifying *string* and *to tighten*, or *to tie with a string*. Galen, from its signification, accepted the word, and from him it has been transmitted through the different epochs of medicine down to our own times. In virtue of its etymological significance, it was formerly applied to any stenosis or closure of duct or aperture, but at present the term is used simply to denote that constriction that affects the prepuce, and which prevents the glans from being passed through the preputial orifice.

Phimosis is said to be congenital or natural and acquired. The first of these is the common lot of all, as a rule, and with some it remains so throughout life. As babyhood advances in boyhood and boyhood into youth, the prepuce gradually becomes lax and distensible, and in proportion to the existence of these conditions it also loses in its length. Where, however, the distal end persists in its constricted condition it is drawn forward as the penis increases in bulk.

In many cases its tightness prevents the escape of the sebaceous matter that collects in the sulcus back of the corona, and the resulting irritation on the surface of the glans and the inner mucous fold of the prepuce ends in an inflammatory thickening of the latter, its inner surface becoming thick, undilatable, hard, and unyielding, all the natural elasticity that should be present having departed, with more or less inflammatory thickening and adhesions between the two layers of skin that form the prepuce.

In this unyielding tube the glans is imprisoned and compressed, often suffering the tortures that the *maiden* of the dungeons of the Inquisition inflicted on the unhappy heretics. It becomes elongated, cyanosed, and hyperæsthetic; the meatus of the urethra is congested and hypertrophied, the corona is undeveloped and often absent, the glans having, on the whole, the long-nosed, conical appearance of the head of a field-mouse. There are hardly five percent of the uncircumcised but who suffer in some degree from this constricting result of the prepuce, to a greater or less extent.

On the other hand, the unconstricted glans penis assumes the shape and appearance that is seen in the circumcised. The head is shorter, the face flat and abrupt, and the meatus, instead of being at the end of a conical point, is situated on the smooth, rounded front of the glans, and does not differ in color from the covering of the glans itself. From the superior commissure of the meatus to the sulcus in the rear of the corona its topographical outline may be said to describe two opposite segments of a circle, as seen in the cuts representing the glans in its natural shape. The corona is prominent and well developed.

The opponents of circumcision base much of their opposition to the fact that circumcision interferes with the natural condition of the parts. The question may well be asked, which of these two shaped glans is the natural product as nature intended it should be? It is a well-known fact that the most forlorn and mouse-headed, long-nosed glans penis will, within a week or two after its liberation from its fetters of preputial bands, assume its true shape.

We may naturally inquire if nature made the glans of a certain shape, which seems to be the proper shape for copulative purposes, only to have the condition most effectually abolished by a constricting, unnatural band? How much the shape of this glans, from meatus to corona, may have to do with retaining the urethra to a healthy and normal calibre and condition has not been inquired into, but, as far as the writer has observed, a normal glans seems to have less abnormalities of the urethra, and in treating such cases he has always found that when the urethra of one of these normal-glans subjects was affected it was far easier to manage; on the other hand, secondary and even a tertiary recurrence to an operation is often the fate of a long, narrow, conical-pointed penis.

Phimosis is known to have been a cause of male impotence by its direct interference with the outward flow of the seminal fluid; but, although we have cases where impregnation has taken place by the aid of a warm spoon and a warm syringe, as in the case related in a former chapter, it must be admitted that the corona is not without some functional office in the act of procreation.

Its shape indicates a valve action like that of the valve in a syringe-piston, and if we examine the two extremes of these conditions of glans—one devoid of corona, as many are, and the other with the corona in its most pronounced form, when in a state of erection—the difference, either in the appearance of the two organs or in the different philosophical action and results that must necessarily follow the use of these two differently shaped glans, will at once be apparent. Unfortunately—or, as many may consider it, most fortunate—the female organs are not always so shaped as to be in themselves wholly favorable to impregnation.

The wearing of corsets, the habitual constipation of females, the relaxed and unnatural condition of the uterine ligaments and vagina in civilized women, all favor uterine displacement, with any or all forms of uterine ailments. To this we may add the effect of repeated miscarriages, application of astringent washes, irregular menstruation, etc., all of which conditions often result in an elongation of the neck, constriction of the cervical canal, with the external os placed on the depended point of the sharply pointed cervix, which is liable to point in any direction.

Just imagine one of these conditioned females and one of the mouse-headed, corona-deficient, long-pointed glans males in the act of copulation! The conical penis finds its way in the reflected fold of the vagina, while the point of the uterus may be two or three inches in some other direction, making impregnation wholly impossible; besides, in the normal-shaped penis, the corona acting as a valve, behind which the circular muscular fibres of the vagina close themselves, tends to retain the seminal fluid in front, while the very shape of the organ assists in straightening out the vaginal canal and to bring the uterus in proper position.

In the long, thin, narrow and pointed glans, devoid

of corona, there is no mechanical means to retain the seminal discharge. Some years ago some one introduced the idea of postural copulation, to be tried in cases of sterility, and it has been found that impregnation would take place in some cases where it had formerly appeared impossible, this position having the effect of righting malpositions during the act, which were the cause of the sterility; but it stands to reason that, where the shape of the organ is such that it further favors malpositions, as well as where it offers no obstacle to the vagina immediately expressing or dropping out all the seminal fluid, impregnation is more difficult, and that, where the uterine deformity is coincident with this condition of penis to assist, it becomes well nigh impossible.

Foderè mentions a penis about the size of a porcupine-quill on an adult male, and Hammond mentions one of the size of a lead-pencil in diameter and two inches in length. From total absence of the penis, either through disease or accident, to the diminutive organs mentioned by Foderè and Hammond, and on up to the full-sized and normal-shaped organ, we have every degree of sizes and shapes, and with these go every conceivable degree of ability or faculty for impregnation.

Aside from the foregoing considerations, there are others equally important. Although Greece was involved for years in war and ancient Troy was destroyed and all its inhabitants slaughtered because of the seduction of one woman; and Semiramis, through her beauty, got all her successive husbands in chancery; and poor, susceptible Samson, from firing Philistine vineyards and killing lions bare-handed, and the Philistines by the thousands with the jaw-bone of an ass, was reduced through Delilah to bitter repentance and turning Philistine mill-stones; and we know that the familiar infatuation of Antony for Cleopatra ruined Antony; and we are familiar with the well-known maxim of the French police-minister, that to catch a criminal it was but necessary to first locate *the woman* and the man would soon be found—society has determined to ignore the influence of the animal passions as factors in our every-day life, or factors in the estrangements, coldness, and the bickerings that end in divorces.

Not to shock the reader with detailed accounts as to what an important factor the shape of the penis may be in the domestic economy, I will refer the reader to Brantome's works.

Although the councils of the older church were not above giving these conditions their calm and deliberate consideration, which resulted in the foundation of the present physical considerations in relation to divorce laws, such studies or considerations are at present only touched upon gingerly and with apologies for doing so, as if the *study of man* was of any less importance to-day from what it was in the days of Moses, the elder church, or when Pope formulated his oft-quoted but little-followed maxim, that *the proper study of mankind is man.*

The present miscalled *delicacy of sentiment* is about as misplaced a condition of disastrous and misleading morality as was the out-of-place and untimely bravery of poor old Braddock when refusing Washington's advice at the Monongahela.

The success and beauty of the Mosaic law is its

squarely facing the conditions of actual life, and its absence from nonsense or nauseating sentimentality. Were our present churches to observe more of this plain talk, for which the good old Anglo-Saxon is as fully expressive and convincing as the old Hebrew, and deal less in rhetorical flourishes and figurative mean-nothings to tickle the ears of our modern Pharisees, mankind as well as womankind would be infinitely so much the better off, mentally, morally, and physically, and there would be less of the conflict between science and religion.

Luther's dream of restoring religion to its primitive purity has come to but as poor realization at the hands of his so-called followers, which leads one to think that if the martyrs of the Reformation could come back and see the fruits of their martyrdom—suffered that pure religion might live—they would conclude that, for all the resulting good accomplished, they might as well have kept a whole skin and a whole set of bones.

In cases of pronounced phimosis the aperture in the prepuce may not be in a line with the meatus, and the resulting discharge of urine or the ejaculations of seminal fluid may from this cause be unable to find an egress.

The fluid escaping from the urethra will, in case the opening is at the side or upper part of the prepuce, cause it to balloon out until a sufficient quantity is thrown out so as to distend, the opening as well as the prepuce, before it can find its way out; in such cases impotency is liable to be as complete as in those cases of stricture wherein the seminal fluid is forced backward into the bladder.

Having given this general view of the effects of phimosis as it may affect man in the shape of his organ, which may have a serious result in his domestic relations or in becoming a father, we will proceed to the consideration of diseases and conditions that phimosis encourages and to which it renders man more liable.

In the consideration of these cases it must not be forgotten that the sexual relations are much more to man or woman than is generally acknowledged. The days for the establishment of the Utopian republic of Plato are not yet with us. That Platonic love does exist is true, as it has in the past and will in the future. Scipio, refusing to accept the beautiful betrothed bride of an enemy as a present, or Joseph leaving his coat-tail in the hands of the amorous bride of the eunuch Potiphar, with the suicide of Lucretia, in the past, are events which virtue and modern continence probably duplicate every day; but these are exceptions to the rule.

Physicians daily see evidences of the most devoted Platonic affection in either sex, but they also see enough of the opposite side of the question to convince them that in the majority of cases the sexual relations are the bond of union, as well as the mainspring of love.

As observed by Montesquieu, the bride of a first-class Turkish eunuch has but a sorry time, and a woman of the same calibre of mind as that possessed by the ordinary Circassian or Armenian bride cannot be in a much happier condition with a husband partly eunuchised by a constricted prepuce.

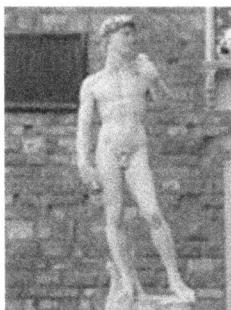

CHAPTER XIX—IS THE PREPUCE A NATURAL PHYSIOLOGICAL APPENDAGE?

By many surgeons the idea of circumcision, unless connected with an immediate demand for interference—such as a phimosis unmanageable by any other means, an induced phimosis from gonorrhoea or other irritation, syphilis in its initiatory sore, cancer or some such cause—is looked upon as an unwarrantable operation, a procedure not only barbarous, painful, and dangerous, but one that directly interferes with the intentions of nature.

The prepuce is by many looked upon as a physiological necessity to health and the enjoyment of life, which, if removed, is liable to induce masturbation, excessive venereal desire, and a train of other evils. The question then resolves itself, what is the real physiological status of this appendage, if it has any, and, if it is a physiological appendage, when does it merge into a pathological appendage?

As by some it is held that the prepuce enjoys the same right to live and exist as the nose, ear, or a limb, which are only subject to amputation in case of a serious disease, they should be reminded that they are not taking into consideration that the nose and ear are calculated to warn us of danger, and that our legs are very useful; as even the great orator Demosthenes, by the timely and rapid use of his legs, was enabled to escape from a battle, where his oratory was of no avail against the illiterate javelins of the unscholarly Macedonians.

If the prepuce only was endowed with an olfactory sense—as, for instance, if a nervous filament from the first pair of nerves had been sent down alongside of the pneumogastric and then, by following the track of the mammary and epigastric arteries, had at last reached the prepuce, where the olfactory sense could have been turned on at will, like an incandescent lamp—it might have been a very useful organ, as in that sense it could have scented danger from afar, if not from near, and enabled man to avoid any of the many dangers into which he unconsciously drops.

But, seeing that the prepuce, to say nothing of being neither nose, eye, nor ear to warn one away from danger, or a leg to run away on after once in it, having not even the precautionary sensitiveness of a cat's moustachios, it cannot, in any way that we can see, be compared to any other useful part of the body.

All attempts to find reasons for its existence that are of real benefit to man have so far proved unsatisfactory, and, unlike the reasons for its removal, are, as a rule, founded on speculation. To further reason out the why and wherefore of its existence or of its summary surgical execution, we must consider its shifting positions as to the effects it produces, as well as to its conditions at different ages, sitting on its case like an impartial jury in the case of some unconvicted but diabolically-inclined criminal.

As before remarked, we are, as a rule, born with this appendage, just as much as we are with the appendix vermiformis, which rises up, like Banquo's ghost, whenever we eat tomatoes or any small-seeded fruit. This prepuce is then long, and the penis is found at the end of an undilatable canal, which is formed by the constricted prepuce; at this early stage of our existence it is often additionally bound down to the glans by a greater or less number of adhesions. We are then in what many term a state of physiological phimosis, that being a perfectly natural condition, and one consistent with health; at least, we imagine it is normal.

Phimosis in childhood is generally considered a physiological state, only to be taken as a pathological condition under certain circumstances. Preputial adhesions may, according to many observers, also be classed as physiological at an early period of life, as it is by them considered as congenital, and common enough to warrant its being classed as normal.

As to the first, or phimosis, it undoubtedly is a physiological condition during infancy; but why, we do not know; and it is also a fact that from birth to puberty it remains so in fully over one-half of the cases. Out of 98 children, from one week to sixteen years of age, examined by Dr. Packard, the prepuce was entirely unretractable in 54, partly so in 3, and wholly so in 36; while in 1 it only half-covered the glans and in 4 the glans was wholly uncovered, 1 of these 4 being an infant only five weeks old.

Dr. Packard also gives the result of 172 examinations by himself, of from twelve to seventy-three years of age, and 106 examinations by Dr. Maury, a total of 278, in whom 100 had a long prepuce, 97 a partly-covered glans, and 81 (of whom 2 had been circumcised) in whom the glans was exposed.[83]

As to adhesions, there is an unaccountable diversity of opinion as to their constancy as a natural condition, being frequent enough to class them as physiological occurrences. Dr. A. B. Arnold, of Baltimore, states that his experience in reference to preputial adhesions leads him to conclude that the frequency of its occurrence has been much overstated. In the number of children that he has circumcised, which exceeds 1000, he has met with it in less than four percent of the cases. He also mentions that in the adult the adhesions show greater firmness.[84]

On the other hand, Dr. Bernheim, of the Paris Israelitish Consistory, observes that, of over 3,000 newborn whom he has examined, with but few exceptions he found the presence of preputial adhesions. He remarks, however, that in the majority these are detached or broken by the first attempt at erection.[85]

Bokai, out of 100 children, found 8 who were over seven years of age, who were perfectly free; while of the remaining 92 under that age 6 more showed no adhesions and 86 had various degrees of adhesions.[86]

---

[83] American Journal Med. Sciences, vol. lx.
[84] *Circumcision*, Dr. A. B. Arnold, of Baltimore.
[85] *De la Circoncision*. By Dr. S. Bernheim. Paris.
[86] The reader is referred to a very interesting paper detailing

Dr. Holgate, of the out-door department of Bellevue, considered that all phimosic cases have adhesions; while Dr. Moses, of New York, out of some fifty circumcisions performed at the eighth day, found only adhesions three times.[87]

These observations are, however, in perfect accord. If we connect the statement of Dr. Arnold, in regard to the increasing character of the firmness in the adhesions of the adult, with the statement of Dr. Bernheim, that the first erection is often sufficient to break up the existing adhesions in the infant, we must conclude that they are nothing more at first than a slight agglutination, which the slight manipulation required to properly locate the position of the glans, and to space out the prepuce preparatory to the operation of circumcision, must, in the majority of cases, be sufficient to liberate the prepuce from the glans; this is evident also from the statement of Dr. Moses, who only found six percent of the cases operated upon by him as being so affected.

The writer has been present at a large number of Hebrew circumcisions performed on the eighth day, and from that up to the sixth month (as in many communities they wait until a number of children are collected, so to speak, before sending for the mohel, who may reside at quite a distance), and in all of those witnessed he has never seen any complications from adhesions; but cases of adhesion have been often

---

conditions of adhesions in the *American Journal Med. Sciences* for July, 1872. It is taken from the Hungarian of M. Bokai.

[87] *New York Med. Journal*, vol. xxvi.

encountered from the second to the eighth year, and it has always been the case, as a rule, that the older the child the greater the firmness of the adhesion.

In these cases the practice generally advised of using a probe is not practicable, as the person is more apt to wound the sound prepuce than to tear the adhesions; the practice most effectual is to hold the glans firmly but gently with the thumb and forefinger of the right hand, and then to draw the prepuce as firmly back with its fold held in the forefinger and thumb of the other. It is a more expeditious mode, and the least painful; by this method extensive adhesions can readily be broken up; vaselin and a piece of fine lint should then be interposed for a couple of days to prevent a re-adherence.

Another co-existing condition with phimosis, very often found, is a shortening of the frenum. Dr. Jansen, out of 3,700 soldiers of the Belgian army, found 12.3 percent with this pathological condition and 2.5 percent with a narrow prepuce.[88]

Take the three conditions above enumerated — phimosis, preputial adhesions, and short frenum—all are but a departure from a normal, in a greater or less degree; and whether the resulting discomfort consists in mere mechanical impediment to urination, erection, or as a factor in nocturnal enuresis, dysuria, impotence, either through reflex action or interference with emission, malposition of the urethral orifice during copulation owing to any of these conditions, or in any of the nervous derangements that may

---

[88] *American Journal Med. Sciences*, vol. lx.

accompany this condition, or in the more serious results, ending in positive deformity of body or limb, or in the warping of moral sentiments, or, even further, in inducing insanity, it cannot well be seen how the conditions that will certainly produce these results, in a more or less degree, can ever, in any logical sense, be considered a physiological condition.

There are certain conditions to life, up to the time of birth, which, unless they then cease at once to exist, immediately become from a physiological into very serious pathological conditions. These are well understood, and have their reasons for existing during our pre-natal existence; but the prepuce has no known function during uterine life or subsequently; and there being no valid reason for its existence, there are certainly no logical grounds for its being considered a physiological condition, especially when the serious results attending the most accentuated form of the above three conditions are considered, and as its necessity, in cases of its entire absence, has not yet been demonstrated.

It can well be said that about two-thirds of mankind are affected in a greater or less degree with these pathological conditions, causing them more or less annoyance. Of these, a certain percentage suffer a life of continued misery, as a direct or indirect result of these conditions.

As to the actual necessity of a prepuce existing, or as to what annoyances or diseases persons are subjected to who are born without it, there is a most singular and expressive silence in medical literature.

It stands to reason that, if it is a necessity, some one person should have found it out long ago, and there should then be some evidence to present in relation thereto. There are cases reported in some of the older surgeries wherein an attempt has been made, in the absence of a prepuce, to restore or manufacture one by means of a plastic operation.

Vidal describes such an operation,[89] but there is no reason given as to why the operation was undertaken; there is no record of any diseased condition which it was intended either to cure or to

---

[89] Dr. Vanier describes this operation of Celsus mentioned by Vidal in his work on *Circumcision*, at page 294, which consisted in making, by a circular incision immediately back of the glans, like in a circular amputation, a complete detachment of the integument from back of the corona. The penis was then made to retreat into the sheath thus made and a short catheter introduced into the urethra, to the end of which the free end of the new preputial fold was made fast, a piece of oiled lint being interposed between the raw inner surface and the glans. Another operation consisted in forcibly drawing the integument forward and in making a number of transverse incisions in the integument so as to assist its extensibility. By these means it was drawn sufficiently forward so as to fasten it to a canula or catheter made fast in the urethra. But it can well be imagined that a person must possess the most exalted idea of the physiological needs of a prepuce and feel the most sensitive need of such an appendage to submit to the first of these operations, although it is more than probable that many Jews submitted to the operation in the days of Celsus to avoid being exiled or plundered of all their possessions. The resulting prepuce could not have been a much more unsightly appendage than that which ornaments the overburdened virile organ of many Christians, and there is no doubt but that in many cases they passed muster.

alleviate; so that we are left to infer that the person simply submitted to the operation from purely cosmetic reasons. The Hebrews of Palestine, after the Roman conquest, or those in Italy or Spain, attempted a like operation, but not from any reason of lessened health or to restore any lacking physiological action, their aim having simply been to hide their identity, for the purpose of escaping persecutions, exactions, or annoyances, either from their rulers or their fellow-citizens.

Dr. A. B. Arnold, in a paper on circumcision, read before the Academy of Medicine of Baltimore, argues that it is not difficult to divine the purposes of the prepuce, holding that it is necessary to protect the tactile sensibility of the glans, due to the presence of the Pacinian bodies which Schweigger Seidel discovered in the nerves, and that a better provision than the anatomy of the prepuce cannot be conceived for shielding the very vascular and sensitive structure of the glans from external sources of irritation and friction, that might rouse the sensibility of this organ, which, on physiological grounds, may cause early masturbation; further arguing that, the corona being undoubtedly the most excitable part of the glans, its denudation by circumcision leaves it more apt to be affected by chance titillations.[90]

In this latter view of the case the preponderance of views is, however, in the opposite direction. J. Royes Bell states that, owing to the induration of the glans through the means of circumcision, masturbation and syphilis are less rife amongst the circumcised than

---

[90] *Circumcision*, Dr. A. B. Arnold.

amongst the uncircumcised.[91]

M. Lallemand, whose experience in the treatment of seminal emissions is of the greatest value, looked upon circumcision as one of the means of curing those diseases, looking on the diminished irritability of the glans resulting from the operation as the curative element.[92]

Dr. Cahen, in a *Dissertation sur la Circoncision*, in 1816, before the Faculty of Medicine of Paris, called the attention to the diminished sensibility of the glans induced by circumcision.

Dr. Vanier, of Havre, looks upon the prepuce as the most frequent cause of onanism.

> *If the prepuce is lax, its mobility produces an irritation to the highly irritable and sensitive nervous system of the child by the titillation in its movements on the glans; if too tight and constricted, then it compresses the glans, and by its irritation it leads the child to seize the organ.*[93]

So that in either case he looks upon the prepuce, through the sensitiveness it retains and induces in the glans, as the principle cause of masturbation. M. Debreyne, the Trappist monk and physician of La Trappe, who has paid considerable attention to medicine as applied to morality, practically makes the same observations.

---

[91] *Int. Enc. Surgery*, vol. vi., Ashhurst.
[92] *Pertes Seminales.*
[93] *Circoncision.* Dr. Vanier, du Havre.

History of Circumcision

In children who have not yet the suggestions of sexual desire imparted by the presence of the spermatic fluid, the presence of the prepuce seems to anticipate those promptings. Circumcised boys may, in individual cases, either through precept or example, physical or mental imperfection, be found to practice onanism, but in general the practice can be asserted as being very rare among the children of circumcised races, showing the less irritability of the organs in the class; neither in infancy are they as liable to priapism during sleep as those that are uncircumcised.

Dr. Bernheim says that:

> *the prepuce may be said in general to be an appendage to man, if not positively harmful in some cases, at least useless, requiring constant care, the neglect of which is liable to entail disease and suffering; the irritation it produces through the sebaceous secretion is a frequent cause of masturbation which nothing short of circumcision will remedy.*

Through middle life, unless the prepuce be the subject of some vicious conformation, little inconvenience may result from its presence, except it be from the dangers to infections already pointed out during this period of life; an ordinarily movable and retractable prepuce will not acquire the condition of phimosis, unless it be through disease or accident; but with our entrance into old age, or after having passed our vigorous prime, the torment of the days of our infancy and childhood come to harass us again.

Persons given to corpulency, with a long prepuce, are apt to become affected with phimosis in their latter years, as such persons are more subject to loss of their sexual vigor and power of erection than lean and spare people; in these, the gradual diminution of the size of the erectile tissues of the organ and its retraction allows of the reconstriction of the preputial opening, which, in the end, will not allow the prepuce to be drawn back over the gland.

These conditions are followed by the irritating affections incident to phimosis of our earlier life, with the modification that age has induced in making us subject to more serious and fatal ailments, both locally and generally.

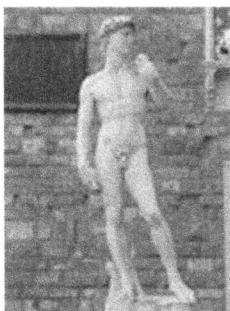

CHAPTER XX—THE PREPUCE, PHIMOSIS, AND CANCER

In the *British Medical Journal* of January 7, 1882, there is an interesting article by Jonathan Hutchinson on the *Pre-cancerous Stage of Cancer*.

In this article he states that, whereas, twenty years previously, his suggestion had been to treat all suspicious sores as being due to syphilis until a clearer diagnosis could be made out, he

> *...had more recently often explained and enforced the doctrine of a pre-cancerous stage of cancer. According to this doctrine, in most cases of cancer, either of penis, lips, tongue, or skin, there is a stage—often a long one—during which a condition of chronic inflammation only is present, and upon this the cancerous process becomes ingrafted. Phimosis and the consequent balanitis lead to cancer of the penis.... A general acceptance of the belief that cancer*

usually has a pre-cancerous stage, and that this stage is the one in which operations ought to be performed, would save many hundreds of lives every year.... Instead of looking on whilst the fire smouldered, and waiting till it blazed up, we should stamp it out on the first suspicion.... What is a man the worse if you have cut away a warty sore from his lip; and, when all is done, a zealous pathologist demonstrates to you that the ulcer is not cancerous, need your conscience be troubled? You have operated in a pre-cancerous stage, and you have probably effected a permanent cure of what would soon have become an incurable disease. I do not wish to offer any apology for carelessness, but I have not in this matter any fear for it.

In view of the great frequency of the occurrence of cancer of the penis, and the facts pointed out by Roux, that, after the removal of the cancerous prepuce or a portion of the penis for cancer, in case of a recurrence the disease does not do so in the penis, but that it attacks the inguinal glands, showing conclusively that the prepuce is the inciting cause as well as the initial point of attack, the sentiments in the foregoing paragraph, taken from the words of Hutchinson, are worthy of our most careful consideration.

M. Roux, Surgeon to the Charité, during the second decade of the present century, first called the attention of the French profession to the intimate relation or dependence that cancer of the penis bears to phimosis. In England he was preceded in this field of surgical investigation by William Hey, whom Roux met in London in 1814. Hey had then operated by amputation of the penis on twelve cases of cancer, nine of whom had had phimosis at the time of the development of the cancer. Wadd at this time also published a work on the subject, but, although he noticed that phimosis was a cause of cancer, he did not fully grasp the subject as Hey and Roux had done, as he believed a cancerous diathesis a primary necessity, and did not then recognize that the primary cause was fully to be found in the prepuce itself.

Roux was probably the first to point out the peculiarly local character of penile cancer, as there is no locality wherein a timely operation is less apt to be followed by a recurrence. He records a number of cases where the prepuce alone was affected when first seen, but none wherein the glans was attacked and where the prepuce was exempt, giving ample evidence of the original starting-point of the disease.[94]

Erichsen also remarks on the little liability to recurrence of cancer of the penis after a timely operation; he divides the cancer to which the penis is subject to as being of two distinct kinds—scirrhus and epithelioma. The latter variety commences as a tubercle in the prepuce, and, according to Erichsen, does not occur in the body of the penis except as a secondary infiltration or deposit.[95][95] Travers states that Jews who are circumcised are not subject to

---

[94] *Dictionaire des Sciences Médicales.*
[95] Erichsen's *Surgery*, page 1144. Edition of 1869.

either form of cancer.[96]

Repeated attacks of herpes preputialis and some consequent point of induration are looked upon by Petit-Radel, Chauvin, and Bernard as frequent starting-points for the cancerous affection of the prepuce. The aged or persons of lax fibre being more subject to these inflammatory attacks, are also the most frequent victims of cancer in this situation. The celebrated Lallemand, in regard to the tendency to cancer induced by the presence of the prepuce, observes as follows:

> *Besides simple balanitis...there also result various indurations, which are proportionate in their degree to the length or time and intensity with which the inciting inflammatory conditions have existed.*
>
> *I have repeatedly found the mucous lining of the prepuce thickened, hardened, ulcerated, and nodulated; at other times converted into a fibrous or even into cartilaginous tissue of excessive thickness; in others, still, in which it had assumed a scirrhous and cancerous nature. I have repeatedly operated on such cases, wherein the prolongation of the prepuce was the only recognized primary cause, the subjects being often countrymen of from fifty to sixty years of age, who had never known any women except their own, but*

---

[96] *Medical News* of Philadelphia, page 115. Vol. for 1860.

who had, nevertheless, been long sufferers
from balanitic attacks, accompanied by
abundant acrid discharges, swellings of
the prepuce, with more or less consequent
excoriations and narrowing of the preputial
orifice.[97]

---

[97] *Pertes Seminales.* In the fourth American edition of the English translation of McDougall of Lallemand we find that he fully appreciated the dangers that lurk in a prepuce. At page 216 he says: "Such is the condition which the parts present in cases of recent balanitis, and these are the inflammations and ulcerations that cause more or less extensive adhesions of the prepuce to the glans. Such adhesions are generally cellular, but sometimes fibrous or even cartilaginous, according to the severity and frequent repetition of the inflammation. Various degrees of induration also results according to the intensity, the duration, and the frequency of the phlogosis. Thus, I have often found a mucous membrane hardened, thickened, and covered with numerous papillæ, sometimes fibrous or cartilaginous, with three times its natural thickness. I have also met with cases in which the prepuce has become cancerous. I have operated in several cases of cancer of the penis, too, which certainly arose from no other cause. The patients were generally peasants between fifty and sixty years of age, who had never known other than their own wives, but who had frequently suffered from balanitis attended by abundant discharge, swelling of the prepuce, and excoriation of its opening, which was so contracted as to prevent the passage of the glans. I have seen one case, also, in which balanitis, irritated by a forced march and the abuse of alcoholic stimulants, passed into gangrene, by which the greater part of the glans was destroyed. Such have been the accidents which I have observed on those

Claparède sums up the inconveniences and dangers to which the possessor of a prepuce is liable to suffer from, as follows:

> *The retention of the sebaceous secretion is liable to alter its character, converting it into an acrid, irritating discharge, which induces more or less burning, smarting, itching, excoriations, and swelling, which, affecting the little glands situated about the corona and sulcus, induces them to secrete an altered and vicious secretion. In this manner a simple elongation of the prepuce will produce an inflammation of the surface of the glans (balanitis), or that of the prepuce itself (posthitis), or the two conjoined (balano-posthitis), complicated possibly with phimosis. By an extension to the mucous membrane of the urethra of the same condition of the inflammatory process, we have blennorrhagia; blennorrhagia is liable to be followed by inguinal swellings or tenderness, orchitis, stricture, and prostatic disease; the formation of preputial calculus, from retention of the urine in the*

---

whose prepuce was too narrow to permit the glans being uncovered; accidents which I can only attribute to the long retention of the sebaceous matter in a kind of *cul-de-sac*, into which a certain quantity of urine passes every time the patient makes water.

prepuce; and cancer is apt to be the end of any of these conditions.[98]

J. Royes Bell, in Ashhurst's "International Encyclopædia of Surgery," observes as follows:

Carcinoma attacking the genital organs usually assumes the form of epithelioma; the other kinds are rarely met with. Epithelioma may invade the prepuce, or the whole penis, or any part of it. The most common age for it is fifty years or over. In the great majority of cases there has existed a congenital or acquired phimosis. A contusion or a urinary fistula may be the exciting cause. With a phimosis the parts are not kept clean, but the gland is macerated and rendered tender and excoriated by retained secretions, and the irritation causes an epithelioma to grow in those predisposed to the disease, as is found to be the case when the tongue is irritated by a broken tooth, or the scrotum by the presence of soot in its folds. Syphilis has no direct influence in inducing the disease, but a syphilitic chap or ulcer may be the starting-point of an epithelioma. Two kinds of epithelioma affect the penis—the indurated and the vegetating, or cauliflower growth.... The nature of the disease, in either the prepuce or the glans,

---

[98] *La Circoncision*, Claparède.

*is masked by a phimosis.... The prognosis
in these cases is much more hopeful than
in epithelioma, in other situations.... Sir
William Lawrence operated on a patient
who was quite well years afterward, and
Sir William Ferguson amputated the penis
of a man of note in the political world, who
lived many years after the operation, and
died at an advanced age.*

Agnew, of Philadelphia, describes an epithelioma of the
prepuce occurring in persons past middle life,
beginning as a tubercle, crack, or wart, for which he
advises an early circumcision; he admits, however, to
not having sufficient data to determine whether Jews
and circumcised persons are exempt from carcinoma
of the penis; but as its usual starting-point he
evidently admits to be in the prepuce, circumcision
must certainly be a preventive to its appearance. Gross
gives substantially the same opinion as Agnew in this
regard. Dr. John S. Billings, in his article on the *Vital
Statistics of the Jews*, in the January *North American
Review*, of 1891, on the subject of cancer, observes as
follows:

*As regards cancer and malignant tumors,
we find that the deaths from these causes
among the Hebrews occur in about the
same proportion to deaths from other
diseases as they do in the average
population. But as the ratio of deaths to
population is less among the Jews, so the
ratio of deaths from malignant diseases to*

population is also less. Among the living population the proportion found affected with cancer among the Jews was 6.48 per 1000, while of those reported sick by the United States census of 1880, for the general population, the proportion was 10.01 per 1000.

There are no convenient data as to the prevalence or percentage of cases of cancer among the Arabian or Mohammedan population of Asia and Africa, but the above comparison of 6.48 per 1000 among the Jews of the United States, against 10.01 per 1000 of the general population, shows that the circumcised race does, in the instance of cancer, certainly enjoy a certain amount of immunity, having in this regard not quite such an exemption as they enjoy from consumption, but still sufficient to assist in making them longer-lived and more able to enjoy life and die a less lingering and painful death.

It is surprising that, in view of the fact that carcinoma of the penis, starting with such frequency in the prepuce, should have left any doubt but that with the absence of this appendage there would follow less liability to cancer. Cullerier informs us that he had several times amputated the penis for cancerous diseases, but that he is unable to tell us whether the persons were affected with phimosis, remarking that on the last case he had observed the indurated remains of the prepuce; he had, however, recognized the necessity of freely exposing the gland in cases where, from continued irritation and inflammation, there was danger of cancer formation.

Nelaton describes two varieties of cancer that affect the penis—that which attacks the integument and that which attacks the glans. The first of these varieties he observes as generally beginning as a hardened nodule in the prepuce, which becomes at once more or less thickened and indurated. He gives Lisfranc the credit of pointing out the fact, that, even in the most hopeless-looking case, the glans and body of the penis may be simply pushed back and compressed, but otherwise sound, and that before resorting to an amputation of the whole organ it is better to make a careful exploratory dissection in search of the penis, as it oftentimes happens that the prepuce and integument can be dissected off, leaving the organ intact. He also mentions that elephantiasis of the penile integument generally begins in the prepuce.

Baron Boyer believed that the vitiated preputial secretion allowed to remain beneath the prepuce was one of the causes of cancer of the penis, observing that it would be interesting to know whether cancer of the penis was a rarity among circumcised people, such as the Jews and Mohammedans.[99]

It is easy to perceive why or how Agnew, Gross, Cullerier, and many of those who have written on the subject, have failed to appreciate the existence of the prepuce as an exciting cause, or as being, in the majority of instances, the part primarily attacked. The nodule, excoriation, or abrasion that develops into a cancer generally produces more or less local disturbance; in many it produces a phimosis that is

---

[99] *Traité des Maladies Chirurgicales*, Baron Boyer. vol. x, page 370.

only relieved by the ulcerative process that exposes the gland, which may by that time itself be attacked or even destroyed. They are then seen by either the rural practitioner or the family physician, but before submitting to an operation they run the gauntlet of many physicians, and, when it comes to operating, they generally apply to some one of great skill and reputation. By this time there is little left of the organ, and, as a rule, the party is unable to tell where the disease originated, whether in the prepuce or glans, to them the swollen prepuce seeming to be the whole organ. Of late years, however, it has been pretty well established that it generally begins in the prepuce, and the great number of amputations of the penis on record for this disease does not lead one to believe that it is as rare a disease as was formerly believed. In Langenbeck's *Archiv*, Bd. xii, 1870, Dr. Zielewicz reports fifty cases of amputation of the penis by the galvano-cautery loop, mostly for carcinoma, one of the fifty being for gangrene and one other for a large papillary tumor. That one surgeon was able to report forty-eight cases of carcinoma or cancer that were treated by one special system of operating tells us plainly enough that the unfortunate possessor of a prepuce, no matter how normal or unobjectionable it may seem to be in the prime of man's existence, or however physiologically necessary it may be deemed, runs too many risks in holding on to his possessions.

The views set forth by Hutchinson in the beginning of this chapter are precisely those that are held by the writer, who would even go further, by advising all such as have, in their youth or since, suffered with balano-posthitis in any degree or form, or whose prepuce shows a tendency to elongation with age, to have the same removed at once; where the prepuce is not redundant, but only tight, a slight operation, such as slitting, will at once remove the possibility of any future danger, without keeping a man from his business a single day.

It may here be remarked that, although always favorably impressed with the great benefits arising out of circumcision, nothing ever resulted in such a serious consideration of the subject as seeing a professional brother dying with a cancerous affection of the penis. The disease had originated in the mucous lining of the prepuce, and when seen in consultation with his attending physicians the gland had already disappeared and the inguinal glands were affected. The man was in the prime of life, and, aside from the local trouble, a specimen of perfect health and physique. He informed us that while a youth he had suffered from repeated attacks of herpes preputialis; that he had suggested circumcision more than once to his father, who also was a physician, but who, unfortunately for the son, could not see any merit in circumcision. To his eyes there was nothing that circumcision could do but what could be accomplished by washing and personal attention to cleanliness. When older, the prepuce gave him less trouble, and for a long time after his marriage it ceased to trouble him altogether. The idea of the necessity of circumcision did not occur to him again until the appearance of the cancerous disease; even then, not appreciating the danger, and looking upon the trouble as a simple transient result of some inflammatory action, he waited until the parts would be in a better state or condition of health before resorting to an operation—that time never came.

Although to Roux, Wadd, and Hey the credit must be given for bringing the subject of cancer of this organ so prominently before the profession, the knowledge of the existence of the disease has long been a matter of record. Patissier, in the fortieth volume of the *Dict. Des Sciences Médicales*, quotes from the third volume of the *Mémoires de l'Académie Royale de Chirurgie*, that in 1724 an officer, aged fifty, was attacked by a cancerous affection originating underneath the prepuce; at the time he consulted MM. Chicoineau and Sonlier the disease had existed for two years, the inguinal glands were implicated, and even the suspensory ligament was affected. These surgeons, nevertheless, determined upon an operation, and, after a long chapter of hæmorrhagic accidents, the patient finally made a recovery. Another case, quoted by Patissier, was operated upon by M. Ceyrac de la Coste, the patient a man of sixty, the disease originating, like the preceding case, underneath the prepuce.

Warren, in his *Surgical Observations on Tumors*, observes that cancer of the penis begins by a warty excrescence on the glans or prepuce.

Walshe, in his work on the *Nature and Treatment of Cancer*, says:

> *The disease may commence in almost all parts of the organ, but the glans and prepuce are by far its most common primary seats. It may originate either from a warty excrescence or a pimple, or it may infiltrate the glans, or appear as a complication of venereal ulceration.*

Peter Charles Remondino

Phimosis, either congenital or acquired, is an exceedingly common accompaniment, and it appears probable that the irritation occasioned by this condition of the parts may act as an exciting cause of the disease in persons predisposed to cancer. Circumcision is, therefore, an advisable prophylactic measure, where the constitutional taint is known to exist.

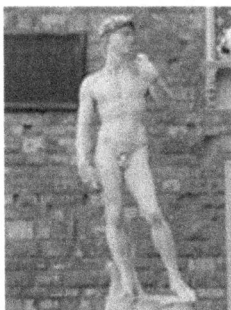

CHAPTER XXI—THE PREPUCE AND GANGRENE OF THE PENIS

Another accompaniment of that preputial appendage is gangrene of the penis, which, like carcinoma, starting in at the prepuce, may invade the pubes and scrotum.

This disease is not so rare as to merit the little attention it has received from our textbooks. M. Demarquay has collected the history of twenty-five cases; from him we learn that the prepuce is the most frequent seat of the start of the affection, from whence, according to Astruc, it rapidly spreads to the skin of the whole organ, and then attacks the corpora cavernosa; it may even extend as high as the umbilicus. This disease spares no age; it attacks young and old alike.

There is not a case recorded of this disease that particularized any other starting-point than the swelling, tension, active or passive congestion that takes place in the integument of the penis. By this it must not be understood that the initial disease or inflammatory action that produces the gangrene must necessarily have its seat in the integument, but that it is the integument of the penis (and especially that of the prepuce) in which, through the laxity of its tissues, passive congestion is favored that the gangrenous action begins.

That this is the actual case there can be but little doubt about, as, even where the gangrene invades the body of the penis itself, even where the inflammatory action may have started from a violent urethritis, that condition of blood which favors gangrenous results will be found to have begun during its state of stasis, where it has parted with much of its watery element, as well as considerable of its vitality, while in its slow, tedious, and obstructed passage through the prepuce.

Some of this dark, thickish blood, finding its way from the integumentary return circulation to that of the deeper structure, becomes there a mechanical as well as a pathological cause for that impediment to the free circulation of the parts, through its altered physiological condition. The deeper structures of the penis, besides their own blood-supply, carry back into the deeper or systemic circulation a large supply from the integumentary tissues, when in the latter, owing to the greater supply due to any inflammatory action, the blood-current is delayed and impeded in its lax and easily-dilatable tissues, and blood-changes occur favoring the gangrene in the deeper tissues, so that, whether the gangrene first takes place in the body of the penis or in the scrotum, it will be in the prepuce or adjoining integument that its real originating causes will be found.

Baron Boyer, in speaking of the inflammation of the penis, observes that the intensity of the swelling, great pain, and difficulty of urination that follow have led many to believe that the inflammation of the deeper structures really always formed a part of the disease.

In otherwise healthy and vigorous subjects it does not, however, extend beyond the skin, as has been demonstrated where the resulting gangrene from excess of inflammatory action has ended in resolution, the deeper tissues not having been found to be injured. It is only where the tone of the general system is lowered, through disease, age, or other deteriorating conditions, that the whole organ is liable to become affected or to break down.

Boyer, in the tenth volume of his *Treatise on Surgical Affections*, gives several examples of this affection not due to age: one case was a person, simultaneously attacked by an adynamic fever and a blennorrhagia, who suffered from gangrene of the penis; the local and constitutional disturbance was not high, however, and the patient escaped with the simple loss of the prepuce.

Another case admitted to the Charité, aged thirty-six, was afflicted with a blennorrhagia, upon which an attack of low fever supervened. The penis inflamed, became engorged and livid, and soon gangrenous symptoms presented themselves, making rapid progress; at first the integument alone was affected, but later all the structures became implicated and the penis was completely destroyed, the sloughs detaching themselves in shreds, leaving a conical stump that healed but slowly.

One case, a young man of twenty, also at the Charité, was admitted with adynamic fever; a few days after admission the prepuce was observed to be somewhat inflamed; in spite of all treatment this progressed so rapidly that the purple discoloration presaged a gangrene, which was not slow in following; the focus seemed to be at the superior and back portion of the prepuce; an incision evacuated a quantity of purulent, serous fluid; the disease, however, extended up the organ as far as its middle before its actions ceased; the sloughs were then cast off, when it was found that part of the gland and a portion of the cavernous body had followed the integument in the general wreck, subjecting the patient to intolerable pain during micturition.

After the recovery from the fever, the remaining portion of the gland and the mutilated parts of the cavernous body were amputated to remedy this condition; the patient subsequently admitted to have had a blennorrhagia at the time of his admission to the hospital.

The gangrenous action may, in proportion to the low condition of the patient, be as proportionately rapid. Another case from Boyer, quoted from the works of Forestus, relates how the whole organ underwent such speedy disorganization that its liquefied remains were found in a poultice, which had been applied with a view of relieving the congestion—a very dear price to pay for retaining the prepuce, that the exquisite sensitiveness of the tactile faculty for enjoyment, resident in the corona of the gland, might not be interfered with.

Gross does not mention this affection in his work on surgery, but Agnew devotes considerable space to its description, dividing the disease into two forms: the inflammatory, such as may follow venereal primary sores or operations on the penis, not excepting circumcision; and the obstructive variety, such as may follow embolism or any mechanical obstruction, either purposely or accidentally applied. Of the latter he gives a number of quoted instances; he only admits seeing one case, that of an aged man in the Pennsylvania Hospital, in whom the disease was caused by embolism of the dorsal artery.

J. Royes Bell, in the *International Encyclopædia of Surgery*, pays more attention to it than any of our American authors; mentioning, among the causes which may give rise to it, the exanthemata, especially small-pox, and the poisoning by ergot of rye and erysipelas. Among the local causes lie mentions phimosis, paraphimosis, and balano-posthitis.

Bell quotes the case reported by Mr. Partridge, in the sixteenth volume of the *Transactions of the Pathological Society of London*, wherein a sober man, aged forty, lost the whole of his penis up to the root, during the course of a typhus fever. Also the case reported by Mr. Gay, in the thirtieth volume of the same *Transactions*, wherein a cabinet-maker, aged thirty-one, lost his penis through the probable results of rheumatic phlebitis, and due to the presence of a plug in the internal iliac vein. In the twelfth volume of the *Transactions* of the same society he finds the record of the case of a soldier who lost his penis through gangrene induced by syphilitic phagedena.

In the consideration of the subject of the prepuce as connected with penile gangrene, it must not be overlooked that the presence of a prepuce may be the inciting cause of some rheumatic affection (the writer has repeatedly seen such), just as such cases are often the result of stricture; as cases of rheumatism that have resisted all remedial means, but that have readily given way to the dilatation of a stricture, are by no means uncommon; not a mere muscular reflex rheumatic pain, but even when accompanied by a rheumatic blood condition.

So that even in such a case as above reported as being due to rheumatic phlebitis, or the case reported in the fortieth volume of the *Dictionaire des Sciences Médicales* by Patissier, wherein a man lost penis and scrotum through gangrene, induced by urinous infiltration, may all in the origin be due, if not to the immediate, to the remote effects of the presence of the prepuce.

In the first volume of *the Journal of Venereal and Cutaneous Diseases* the writer reported a case of the complete loss of penis in a young man as a result of phagedena due to syphilis. The man had had a long and pendulous prepuce; in his case, had circumcision been performed in early childhood, it would have lessened the chances of primary infection, and had it been performed after his infection, it would have removed one cause—if not the principal cause—of the ease with which the phagedenic action was inaugurated.

The case already mentioned as an example of spontaneous and natural circumcision belongs to the gangrenous results following phimosis, ending with the loss of the prepuce. In Maclise's *Surgical Anatomy* several specimens of deformity are figured, showing the results of this mildest of the effects of a phagedenic action. The beginning of the interference in the return preputial circulation undoubtedly always takes place over the superior aspect of the corona, where the pressure of the glans is most sharply defined against the inner fold of the prepuce.

There are milder conditions, wherein the circulation of the prepuce is materially interfered with, both through the lax tissues of the parts and the peculiar anatomical construction and shape of the neighboring parts, wherein, without going as far as gangrenous breakdown, the person suffers considerably nevertheless, and is placed in danger of losing his penis; for, as observed by Patissier, whenever a person affected with a gonorrhoea is attacked by a putrid or any low-grade fever, he runs the greatest danger of losing his virile member through gangrene.

Even where phimosis does not exist, but only the long, lax, and retractable prepuce, that is considered a perfectly physiological condition, the prepuce is liable to cause very distressing and complicating annoyances during the progress of other diseases. The writer has noticed that cases with a thick, leathery, and redundant prepuce, even when perfectly retractable, are more liable to require the use of the catheter during the course of a continued fever. Such a condition is also a very frequent accompaniment of prostatic obstruction.

So often has this been noticed that its association with prostatic trouble or disease tends to the belief that the irritation produced by this condition of prepuce often lays the foundation for prostatic disease in not a few cases.[100] In elderly people, with the atrophied penis and elongating prepuce, the constant moisture from the urine on the inner fold and glans adds greatly to the irritation as well as to the discomfort of the patient.

A number of affections are accompanied by oedema, especially toward the latter stages of the disease; such, for instance, as the ending of cases of mitral insufficiency. In these, the distension of the prepuce and the resulting balano-posthitis is at times a source of great distress, and at times the resulting engorgement produces a retention of urine.

It was after an attendance on one such case that required daily and frequent puncturings for its relief, but which, in spite of all care, finally became gangrenous, that a fellow practitioner cheerfully submitted to circumcision, to avoid the possibility of any such complication occurring to embitter his closing illness.[101]

---

[100] I have practiced considerably among the Jewish people, but I have never seen their elderly men suffer with prostatic troubles like our own people who are uncircumcised. From having observed the tendency to prostatic complications in young people with troublesome prepuces, and that the great number of the elderly people who are affected with prostatic disease or enlargement are the unlucky possessors of long or large prepuces, I have arrived at the conclusion that the prepuce can be entered as a factor in the etiology of enlarged prostate.

[101] I have now under my care a poor consumptive who has all the appearance of having always been as virtuous as Joseph, but who, unlike Joseph, has from infancy had as a

History of Circumcision

The prepuce is the starting-point of many of the cases of penitis and retention of urine that often accompany attacks of gonorroea; especially can this result be anticipated where the prepuce is long, pendulous, and with its veins in a varicose condition.

---

constant companion a long, miserable, smegmanous, and annoying prepuce.

The young man has an oedema which first affected his feet, but one day, owing to the irritation of a slight balanitis, the prepuce swelled at once; it proceeded through the penis integument to the scrotum; the penis itself retracted, leaving the integument and scrotum to assume a translucent, puffy, cork-screw appearance and attitude; from its labyrinthic passage the urine slowly dribbles during urination in a scalding stream. In addition to the physical sufferings, he is tormented by the knowledge that his friends attribute all his disease and troubles—since the occurence of the penile oedema—to the fact that his earlier manhood must have been indiscreet, as well as sinful. The laity cannot connect any penile, scrotal, or testicular disease with anything except venereal disease; and if the physician attempts to explain matters, they simply look upon it as the good-natured and well-intentioned efforts of the doctor to deceive them and to cover up the shortcomings of some frail mortal. Many a poor fellow has to leave this world under a cloud of mistrust and a bad odor of past deviltry to which he is not entitled, and suffer all this in addition to all his physical ills, owing to his having been ornamented through life with an annoying prepuce— the luckless heritage of having been born a Christian. Columbus in chains moralizing on the ingratitude of this world is nothing to the poor invalid with a swollen prepuce, innocently acquired, silently "cussing" the ignorance of his relatives and friends.

Why it should be so is self-evident.

Anything that will add to the interference of the return circulation only exaggerates the tendency to penis engorgement; this increases the difficulty of urination, which, by the retention that results, in turn increases the constriction at the root of the penis, and adds to the already difficult return circulation. The bladder by its urine, and the penis by its blood, actually form, by their mutual pressures, an impassable dam at the root of the organ. That this is the true condition has been more than once verified from the instant relief given to the whole condition by the prompt employment of the supra-pubic puncture or aspiration, as catheterization in such cases is altogether out of the question, and should never be attempted or employed unless a soft catheter can be inserted.

A person laboring under a continued fever has his blood in a condition to favor sphacelus; with the slow-moving current of vitiated blood and its retention in such lax tissues as those of the prepuce, through the medium of the enlarged preputial veins, coupled with the lessened sensibilities of the bladder and his perhaps semi-conscious or unconscious condition, and an equally unconscious bladder, he is, to say the least of it—if in possession of a prepuce—also the unconscious possessor of a certain degree of percentage, no matter how small or fractional that may be, of recovering from his fever without his penis.

Dr. W. W. McKay, of the U. S. Marine Hospital Service of San Diego, attended a case of typho-malarial fever in consultation with me, where, but for the persistent, intelligent, but delicate use of the catheter for nearly three weeks the penis would have become gangrenous. The subject was an uræmic, irritable, nervous, leathery-prepuced individual; the organ was unusually large, the skin of the penis thick, and it was only by keeping the bladder empty that prevented a state of engorgement that would have effectually interfered with further catheterization. As it was, the penis was often dank, livid, and discolored from the passive engorgement.

The writer saw a similar case with the late Dr. F. H. Milligan, of Minnesota. The congestion in this case was due to a gonorrheal inflammation involving the skin of the whole penis, retention having followed painful micturition, and the swelling of the penis following the retention; the prepuce was enormously distended, and the penis seemed in a state of erection as far as dimension and rigidity were concerned.

The man, a steam-boat cook, informed us that it was fully twice as large as when rigidly erect in health. All efforts to reduce the swelling were unavailing; neither punctures, leeches, nor scarifications were of any avail; catheterization was impossible, but, after relieving the bladder by the supra-pubic aspiration, the patient experienced some relief. He, nevertheless, lost the whole skin of the penis, with that of the pubis and on the front of the scrotum.

The man ran into a low form of fever, with uræmic symptoms; the stench was so great that it was almost impossible to remain in the same room with him; but he finally made a slow and very tedious recovery. In healing there was considerable downward curvature of the penis, which, however, did not prevent him from following his old, dissolute course of life.[102]

A calm, unprejudiced consideration of the subject of the liability of the uncircumcised races dwelling in the temperate and semi-tropical countries to cancer, gangrene, and elephantiasis might well lead one to ask: Why are we afflicted with a prepuce? We can understand how a man may become gouty, and become a subject in the end for a gangrene of the extremities; or how senile gangrene may, through a series of pathological processes and blood changes, with the aid of age, finally be reached; or how, by a like course of diseased processes, we reach the apoplectic stage.

These conditions, however, can be put off, or partly, if not wholly avoided, by a proper course of life, and, at the worst, it is only after the fires of our youth and prime have completely burned out, that these conditions are liable to claim us as their lawful victim. Not so, however, with some of these conditions that

---

[102] This patient, on convalescing, suffered considerable from the action of numerous small carbuncles, resulting from the toxæmic condition induced by the partial suppression of urine that he at times suffered from, and, when nearly well, brought on a serious relapse by the mail-bag appendage at the penis working up the organ into a state of erection. While so situated he had intercourse, and from 99° his temperature immediately rose to 104½°, where it remained for several days, lengthening out his illness by several weeks, into a long-protracted convalescence. The man is not yet circumcised, and, from the knowledge that I have of his tendency to uræmia, I feel that, although in his prime, a fever or an accident may take him off at any moment.

may end in penile gangrene; that are liable to pounce upon us unawares, like an Apache in an Arizona cañon; or as the hired mercenaries of old Canon Fulbert did upon poor Abelard in his study, and, without further ado or ceremony emasculate man as effectually as the most exacting Turk could demand, with a veritable *taillè à fleur de ventre* operation.

Nature has her own ways of protecting what there is of any utility; there is a law of the survival of the fittest that we all appreciate. If, then, this penile appendage is of any utility, why is it that, unlike the rest of the body, it falls such an easy victim to gangrene?

The procreative function seems to be, in a sense, one of the main cares of nature in its relation to the animal as well as the vegetable kingdom; but here is a useless bit of skin, adipose tissue, mucous membrane, and some connective tissue, that on the least provocation is liable to go off into a gangrene and drag one of the main generative, or even all the procreative, apparatus into the general wreck.

Nature certainly never intended anything of the kind. To be generous, and not libel nature, we must conclude that the prepuce is a near relative to the fast-disappearing climbing-muscle; very useful in our primitive, arboreal days, when we needed such a muscle to reach our perch for the night, and a prepuce or something of the kind, in default of a breech-cloth, to protect the glans penis from being scratched by the briars or thorny and rough bark of the trees in our ascent.

The prepuce was well enough in our primitive and arboreal days—ages and ages ahead of our cave and lake dwellings—when the notch in a tree and its rough bark formed our couch; but in these days of plush-cushioned pews and opera-seats, cosy office-chairs, car-seats, and upholstered furniture or polished-oak seats, it serves no intelligent purpose.

Emasculation has never been looked upon with favor by its victim, and it would be but natural to suppose that man would take every precaution against the accidental occurrence of such an undesired condition.

The writer well remembers that, in his *Tom Sawyer* days on the banks of the upper Mississippi, in the happy days of the crack rafting crews, before the introduction of the towage steamer, when the river towns were more or less terrorized by wild gangs of these men, some of whom were always fighting and quarreling and drinking when not at work.

In the lot there was one man with a great reputation at a rough-and-tumble fight. His main hold was that he generally tried to emasculate his adversary by destroying the physiological condition of the testicle. The man was not a large or powerful man, nor was he a great boxer or wrestler, but this reputation made him feared by all the bullies on the river.

The report that not a few who had tackled him had subsequently been of no value, either as fornicators or fecundators, or had to be castrated on account of the resulting testicular degeneration, seemed in no way to encourage any one to wish to meet him in a personal encounter. It would seem as if the desire to avoid such an accident—provided persons knew the dangers that lurk in a prepuce—would induce many to submit to circumcision.

That many more do not do so can only be attributed to the general human wish to escape a less present evil for a greater unknown one, being evidently deterred by the prospective pain that must be suffered immediately.

There is a question that should interest man above that of the simple loss of penis. It appears that there is a powerful moral effect that follows this loss, as might, in the majority, be anticipated.

According to the experience of Civiale, many who have lost the penis, through amputation for disease or through disease itself, end in suicide. He mentions particularly a patient at the Charité who had lost his penis, who, finding no other means to take himself off, saved up sufficient opium, from that given him to calm his pains, to take all at one dose and commit suicide. In the London *Lancet* for March 27, 1886, there is reported a discussion on this subject, to which the reader is referred, as it fully covers the moral and physical effects of castration and penis amputation for disease.

M. Roux, who amputated the penis of a brother of Buffon, in 1810, reported that, in that case, M. Buffon lost none of his customary gayety.

Peter Charles Remondino

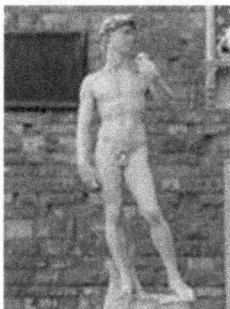

CHAPTER XXII—THE PREPUCE, CALCULI, AND OTHER ANNOYANCES

From an article published in the New York *Medical Times* of March, 1872, from the pen of Dr. J. G. Kerr, of Canton, China, we learn that phimosis is not an uncommon occurrence among the Chinese.

As has been demonstrated by C. H. Mastin, of Mobile, climate is a great factor of calculus.[103] That of China seems a most favorable climate in this regard; so that, between the prevalence of phimosis among the Chinese and the calculus-producing tendency of the climate, China may be said to be the classic land of preputial calculi, as England is that of the gout, or the United States that of delirium tremens.

From Dr. Kerr we learn that the occurrence of these concretions were, as a rule, multiple, and that in two cases that fell under his observation the number of stones from each individual exceeded one hundred. In one case there were forty, and in three cases there

---

[103] *Transactions International Medical Congress* of 1876, page 609.

were between twenty and thirty. These were of different sizes and weight, some being an inch and five-eighths in diameter, and from that size down to where one hundred and sixteen taken from one individual case only weighed one ounce.

The tendency to calculous disease in that climate may well be imagined, when the same observer relates a case of urinary infiltration into the skin on the under side of the penis that gave rise to the formation of a collection of calculi in that locality, four of which were the size of pigeons' eggs; and another case in which a urinary fistula induced the formation of a calculus in the groin, near the scrotum, the calculus weighing two and a half drachms and measuring one and a half inches by three-quarters of an inch in diameter.

Claparède mentions a case in the practice of M. Dumèril, in which the stone extracted from the prepuce weighed two hundred and twenty-five grammes, or about eight ounces.

Civiale speaks of a young man of twenty with phimosis, who, after practicing sexual connection for the first time, experienced pain and a purulent discharge, from whom, on examination, he removed five stones as large as prunes. The patient had felt them in their position, but had imagined the condition to be a natural one.

E. L. Keyes gives their composition as being of calcified smegma, urate of ammonium, triple and earthy phosphates and mucus, and as symptoms and results: pain, purulent discharges, interference with urination and the sexual act, involuntary emission, ulceration of the preputial cavity, and impotence.

Enoch mentions a child of two years in the Charité,

who, being operated upon for phimosis, was found to have a preputial calculus occluding the urethral meatus. At the autopsy a calculus as large as an egg was found in the bladder.

The presence of these formations, although not necessarily dangerous in themselves, may, by their effects and in the irritation they induce, be the means of producing serious mischief. The only preventive or remedy for this condition is circumcision.

Acquired phimosis has been mentioned as a result of inflammatory lotion, such as is connected with balano-posthitis; it sometimes happens that, the act of coitus being done forcibly, especially with public women, who are apt to use very astringent and constricting washes, the prepuce becomes injured, with the result of producing a phimosis.

One man will produce the same results through the means of some vaunted wash or dip which is supposed to act as a prophylactic to any venereal infection. One patient had developed a chronic herpetic affection by the constant use of an iodized ointment which he regarded as an infallible prophylactic. Many cases of phimosis result from the attending inflammation that follows on the liberal domestic application of nitrate of silver to an abrasion after connection, in the mistaken idea that the party labors under, that he is destroying some venereal virus.

By the irritation that all these applications and accidents induce, warts and vegetations are the but too frequent results. These I have never seen in a circumcised individual, and their occurrence and frequency, as well as persistency, are directly proportionate with the degree of tightness, thickness, or redundancy of the prepuce and the irritability of the gland.

As remarked by Lallemand, in reference to the victim of nocturnal enuresis becoming a future victim of nocturnal emissions, so it may be said of the person subject in early life to either warts, excoriations or vegetations on the penis, that it is this class that furnishes in after life the subjects for cancerous disease as well as furnishing the easiest victims for venereal infection. These warts, although easily removed, have a tendency to recurrence, especially as long as the moist bed that has once grown them there is still vegetating.

The prepuce is liable to indurations and hypertrophy. Of the first anomaly, the London *Lancet* of 1846 has a record of two cases in which paraphimosis was induced in elderly subjects, and of one in which it induced phimosis.

Since then a number of cases of thickening and induration have been reported. Hypertrophy may take place in any degree, varying from the mere leathery and overpendulous but unobstructive prepuce to the case recorded by Vidal, in the fifth volume of his *Pathologie Externe et Médecine Operatoire,* which happened in the practice of M. Rigal, de Gaillae.

The hypertrophied prepuce was something enormous, and hung down to below the patient's knees; it was pear-shaped, with the base hanging downward; this base was as large as a man's head. This prepuce was successfully removed by M. Rigal, who presented the specimen before the Paris Surgical Society, who were then discussing a somewhat similar but not so extensive a case, presented by M. Lenoire.

Vidal mentions having operated on a number of cases of this deformity of the prepuce in various degrees of growth.

As a rule, simple hypertrophic disease of the penile integument does not interfere with the sexual functions of the male organ after its removal; it being susceptible of complete removal in exaggerated cases, even without touching the body of the organ.

There are exceptions to this rule, however, when even this otherwise non-malignant disease may entail the loss of all the genitals. In the London *Lancet* of July 11, 1846, at page 46, there is a record of a remarkable case of this nature reported by F. H. Brett, Esq., F.R.C.S. The case was that of a locksmith of forty years of age, who was naturally much phimosed.

The penis was enormously enlarged, as well as the scrotum, which was more or less ulcerated and full of sinuses filled with a serous pus; some six months prior to the final operation, a part of the prepuce was removed to facilitate urination, but the whole mass had to be subsequently removed, including the whole of the skin of the penis and the scrotum, the testicles having been carefully dissected out and recovered with some skin flap.

In this case the disease was believed to have originated from a perineal fistula. The pathological investigation in the case, however, by Mr. Quekett, who submitted the mass to a microscopical examination, confirmed Mr. Brett in his original opinion that the disease had the same pathological conditions as the similar disease found in India, where it originates from local inflammatory causes.

In this case the preputial irritation was, in all

probability, the precursor of the conditions that led to the perineal fistula, the patient having had a stricture for some twelve years. Mr. Brett states that the man had been abandoned by his wife on account of his previous sexual disability, and on account, as well, of his having been incapacitated from following any vocation. After the operation all his functions were restored and his organs were sound.

Nelaton records a case reported by Wadd, in 1817, of an African negro so affected, whose penis measured fourteen inches in length and twelve and a half inches in circumference; also the case reported by Gibert, of Hospital St. Louis, of a subject "with a penis the size of a mule's."

Mr. Brett attributes the recovery of his case as being due in a great measure to the moral support given to the patient from the knowledge that his procreative organs were not interfered with, and on the same grounds he attributes the great fatality previously attending the operation to the fact that it previously had been the custom in many cases to make a clean general *taillè à fleur de ventre*, sacrificing all the genital organs.

In simple hypertrophy, he considers that the body of the penis and the testicles will always be found to be in a normal condition; a careful dissection of the parts will invariably save not only the man's sexual functions, but his moral stamina, which he sadly needs in such an emergency.

In the discussion on this subject heretofore mentioned as taking place in the London Medical Society, Mr. Pye, Mr. John A. Morgan, and others insisted on the necessity of retaining the testicles, whenever possible, in all these sweeping operations upon the genitals, they being actually necessary for the moral and physical support of man, Mr. Morgan observing that their removal would depress parts controlled by the sympathetic system.

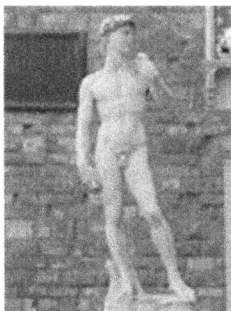

CHAPTER XXIII—REFLEX NEUROSES AND THE PREPUCE

We have seen in the previous chapters what the immediate effects of the prepuce may lead to; we have followed its local effects in childhood to youth, thence into what it does in our prime, and we have seen how, when we are on the down grade, owing to the increase of years, then, like the minute-men of Concord, wakened up by Paul Revere's classic ride, hanging on to the rear of the retreating and disheartened British, it harasses, worries, and downs a man here and there, striking down the man as if it had some undying, irremediable spite, which nothing but his misery and death could alleviate.

Some authorities will argue that all that is required is cleanliness; that all men need do is to be like a true American, with the old Continental watchword of "eternal vigilance is the price of liberty" in continued active practice.

A bowlful of some antiseptic wash and a small sponge should always be at hand, and he should be as

329

industrious as if haltered in a tread-mill; he should make this a part of his toilet, and his daily and hourly care. This will, we are told, lessen his chances of becoming a victim to the many ills that lie in wait for him, all on account of the glory, honor, and comfort of wearing a prepuce, which is a perfectly physiological appendage.

From these visible and apparently easily understood conditions and results we are now to enter a broad field, wherein the prepuce seems to exercise a malign influence in the most distant and apparently unconnected manner; where, like some of the evil genii or sprites in the Arabian tales, it can reach from afar the object of its malignity, striking him down unawares in the most unaccountable manner; making him a victim to all manner of ills, sufferings, and tribulations; unfitting him for marriage or the cares of business; making him miserable and an object of continual scolding and punishment in childhood, through its worriments and nocturnal enuresis; later on, beginning to affect him with all kinds of physical distortions and ailments, nocturnal pollutions, and other conditions calculated to weaken him physically, mentally, and morally; to land him, perchance, in the jail, or even in a lunatic asylum.

Man's whole life is subject to the capricious dispensations and whims of this Job's-comforts-dispensing enemy of man.

As strange as it may seem, this field of knowledge, this field of misery and suffering, disease and distortion, of physical and mental obliquity, presided over by this preputial Afrit of malignant disposition, was an unknown, undiscovered, and therefore unexplored region for some thousands of years, and it remained for an American to discover and describe this vast territorial acquisition, and to annex it to the domain of medicine, which, through its skill, could modify the influence of the evil genius that there presided and spare humanity much of the ills to which it had been subjected.

In this regard, Louis A. Sayre was to medicine what Columbus was to geography. Neither Strabo nor Herodotus had anything to say regarding what existed beyond the pillars of Hercules, and neither Hippocrates nor Galen had anything in regard to this preputial Merlin, which in their day, even, had its existence.

Neither did Tissot nor Bienville, the two pioneers in the field of our knowledge regarding onanism and nymphomania, dream of the existence of this one cause of the diseases to which they gave so much time and study.

It is only some twenty years since Louis A. Sayre read his paper, entitled *Partial Paralysis from Reflex Irritation Caused by Congenital Phimosis and Adherent Prepuce*, before the American Medical Association. This was the starting-point from whence the profession entered into what had previously been a veritable *Darkest Africa*.

When we read that only some fifty years before the times of Columbus Christian Europe had no lunatic asylum—not that there was a lack of lunatics or that the existence of lunacy was entirely ignored, but that the then state of medicine and the general intelligence was not emancipated from the idea of demoniacs—and we are told that the lunatics were in many instances hung, quartered and burned, hooted and chased about the streets, or chained in gloomy dungeons; until, as related by Lecky, a Spanish monk named Juan Gilaberto Joffe, filled with compassion at the sight of the maniacs who were hooted by crowds through the streets of Valencia, founded an asylum in that city.

His movement in this direction called the attention of the Church and people to this class in a practical light, and from Spain a more enlightened idea in regard to this class swept onward throughout Europe. As observed, it seems strange to us of the present day that such ignorance in these matters should, or could, have so long existed.

It seems impossible for us to conceive how these conditions of incoherent action and of mental derangements could have existed and their causes have not been fully appreciated; and yet we were not above, some twenty years ago only, subjecting children to punishment and scoldings for being addicted to nocturnal enuresis, or of accusing cases of nocturnal and involuntary emissions as being due to masturbation. The child was allowed then to grow up paralytic, or with a deformed limb, or continually punished to correct what was imagined to be a condition of willful carelessness, irritability, or willful moral perversion.

Perversion, stupidity, and irritability of the mind or temper were not known to depend, in many instances, on preputial irritation; children were, accordingly, worried and punished for something over which they had no earthly control or the least volition. Humanity cannot, at present, sufficiently appreciate what Louis A. Sayre has done in its behalf. It is here that we realize the hidden wisdom of the Mosaic law and the truth of the assertion of the late Dr. Edward Clarke, that,

> *The instructors, the houses and schools of our country's daughters, would profit by reading the old Levitical law. The race has not yet outgrown the physiology of Moses.*

These irritations from the preputial irritability are not always so slow moving as to span over either months or years in their fell work. Instances of their sudden action have been sufficiently recorded as to warrant them as being classed as causative agents in acute affections that instantly threaten life.

In the London *Lancet* of May 16, 1846, there is a record of a very peculiar case reported to the London Medical Society by Dr. Golding Bird:

> *The case was that of a child seven or eight weeks old only, an out-patient of Guy's Hospital. The child had become almost lifeless immediately after nursing, and to all appearances looked as if under the influence of some narcotic. It had not, however, had anything of the kind given to it, nor had it sustained a fall, nor was the head so large as to lead to suspicion of congenital hydrocephalus. On inquiring if the child passed water, the answer led to an examination of the prepuce, which was found to be elongated, and had an aperture only of the size of a pin-hole, like a*

puncture in the intestines. The urine was dribbling out; it was evident that the child had never completely emptied its bladder. Mr. Hilton slit up the prepuce, and all the symptoms were immediately relieved and soon entirely removed.

Dr. Bird referred to a case which he had related to the Society some years before, which was reported in the *Lancet* at the time, of a child who fell a victim to a malformation of this kind, and after death the bladder and ureter were found like those of a man who had long suffered from stricture.

Mr. Hilton has seen many cases similar to the one mentioned by Dr. Bird. The greatest benefit resulted from slitting up the prepuce. In this case the benefit was very remarkable, a partial paralysis of the left side, under which the little patient labored, being quite removed in twenty-four hours.

In this case the difficulty was evidently both the result of mechanical pressure and reflex irritation. A somewhat similar case as to its results is given by Dr. Sayre, to whom the case was reported by Dr. A. R. Mott, Jr., of Randall's Island, in January of 1880:

John English, aged 46, native of England, widower, clerk; admitted to workhouse hospital. Patient had been at work for a week as a prisoner; on the 23d of December was noticed to be restless and uneasy, and finally, in the evening, he fell from his bunk in a fit. During the next forty-eight hours he had several convulsions, and during the intervals lay in a semi-comatose condition, showing no consciousness except to stir a limb when pinched. Pulse, 120; temperature, 101½°; respiration, 18. Swallowed nothing, and passed fæces in bed. Continued in this condition until December 25th (temperature having fallen to 100°), when a string was discovered passed twice around the penis behind corona and tied, the long prepuce serving to conceal it from observation. While not sufficiently tight to occlude the urethral canal, still a firm, indurated band remained after the string was cut, and did not disappear for four or five days.

Within one hour after the removal of the string the man sat up and asked for milk, and from this time remained perfectly well (was under observation for three months). He declared that he remembered nothing that had taken place during the past three days; had never had fits, denied venereal diseases, was moderately addicted to drink, but had led a 'virtuous life since the death of his wife, two years before.'

The following case in the practice of Dr. F. J. Wirthington, of Livermore, Pa., was also reported to Dr. Sayre:

When the child was born, he was considered the biggest and finest boy that had been born in the community for a long time, until, when he was about two and a-half years old, and being sick, a doctor was called in, who told them that their child was paralyzed, the paralysis being in his lower extremities, and who treated him with the usual nerve-tonic and with electricity.

Notwithstanding all this, the boy went steadily down, and the paralysis continued until he was seen by Dr. Wirthington. The child was then unable to walk; on examination, the prepuce was found to be adherent almost all the way around the glans penis. Behind the corona was a solid cake of sebaceous matter. The case was promptly operated upon, and, although the previous attendant had not found any cause to account for the paralysis, a rapid recovery took place, the boy being able to walk even before the complete cicatrization of the wound, and was soon the picture of health.

Dr. T. F. Leech, of Attica, Fountain County, Ind., reports a case of a fourteen-month-old child, who had been the terror of all that part of the town for over six months, as he cried constantly. Except when asleep or nursed by his mother, he would lie perfectly still and squall, not showing any disposition to sit up; nor did he like to be raised up. He was very nervous, and would have times when his limbs would be rigid. This state of things grew worse, until the child was accidentally seen by Dr. Leech, who, on examination, found a contracted and adherent prepuce, the child being at the time in a high fever and suffering great nervous excitement. An operation by slitting and breaking up the adhesion afforded immediate relief; the spinal irritation, partial paralysis of the lower extremities, spasms during urination, and all trouble disappeared as if by magic.

Prof. J. H. Pooley, of Columbus, Ohio, reported the case of a fine, healthy boy who, up to three months before being seen professionally, had always been well and in perfect health. His condition was found by Professor Pooley to be one of localized chorea, manifesting itself in constant convulsive movements of the head. They were nodding or antero-posterior movements, alternating with lateral or shaking and twisting motions; these movements had become almost constant during the waking hours of the child.

There was no distortion of the features nor any choreic movements of the extremities; indeed, the whole affection consisted in the nodding and shaking movements of the head referred to. These were almost incessant, sometimes slow and almost rhythmical, then for a minute or two rapid and irregular, seeming to fatigue the little fellow, and accompanied by a fretful, whimpering cry.

The child had been subjected to a variety of treatment, but without any benefit or effect of any kind. Upon the most careful examination of the patient and his history, Professor Pooley could not discover anything that seemed to throw any light upon the case, except a condition of well-marked phimosis. Acting upon this, the Professor immediately circumcised the child, and from the very day of the operation the spasmodic action began to diminish, and in two weeks he was entirely well, without any other treatment of any kind.

Dr. W. R. McMahon, of Huntington, Indiana, has reported three cases of epilepsy in children caused by congenital phimosis that were entirely relieved by an operation without any subsequent return of the difficulty. One of the cases was in a boy ten years old, with very firm preputial adhesions and a high grade of inflammation of the parts.

Dr. J. D. Griffith, of Kansas City, Mo., operated on a case of phimosis on a child nearly three years of age, who was afflicted with repeated attacks of convulsions and paralysis of the hips and lower extremities; the little fellow had as many as fifteen convulsions in a day; the patient was greatly troubled with painful urination and priapism. On examination at the operation, a firmly adherent prepuce and a large roll of caseous matter was found just back of the corona. A complete recovery followed the removal of these conditions.

The above cases are taken from the paper read before the Section of Diseases of Children at the International Medical Congress of 1887, by Dr. Sayre. It contains a number of additional cases of an analogous character to the above, reported to him by physicians in different parts of the country.

They show the variety, extent, and far-reaching character of the diseases induced by any preputial irritation. Dr. G. L. Magruder, of Washington, D. C., in the same paper, has a record of twenty-five cases of various nervous disturbances which he had entirely relieved by circumcision or dilatation, without any medication whatever. Dr. Magruder, in concluding his report, in which he quotes the authority of Brown-Séquard, Charcot, and Leyden, as having noticed serious nervous disturbances resulting from reflex irritation due to affections of the genito-urinary organs, observes as follows:

> *From the foregoing, I think that we are justified in the conclusion that phimosis and adherent prepuce give rise to varied troubles of more or less gravity, manifesting themselves either in the muscular, osseous, or nervous systems; and that the removal of these abnormal conditions of the penis frequently affords marked relief, and, at times, perfect and permanent cure.*

In the discussion that followed the reading of Dr. Sayre's paper, Dr. De Forest Willard, of Philadelphia, remarked that he had operated by simply stripping back the prepuce and that he did not circumcise, but that he looked upon the subsequent cleanliness of the parts as the greatest safeguard, not only as against reflex irritation, but also against masturbation.

Retained filth and smegma are far more likely to call a boy's attention to his penis by their unrecognized irritative effects than washing can possibly do. His practice is in accordance with the belief that young children can be relieved by the simpler methods, such as dilatation; but he also observes that when a child has reached eight or ten years of age, and has never been able to expose the glans, contraction is almost certain to be present, and circumcision must be performed. In adults there is rarely any escape when the prepuce is tight.

Dr. I. N. Love, of St. Louis, said:

> *It has been my judgment and my practice for many years, in these reflex irritations, to pursue the radical course of circumcision. I believe thoroughly in the Mosaic law, not only from a moral but also from a sanitary stand-point. All genital irritation should be thoroughly removed. It is all very well to instruct the mother or the nurse to keep the parts within the prepuce clean, but they can not or will not do it. Complete and proper removal of the covering to the glans takes away all the cause of disturbance. Dr. Sayre takes a more pronounced position on this subject than the majority of those who have discussed his paper. An improper performance of a surgical procedure is no argument against the operation, but rather against the operator. For the reasons I have given, I am in favor of the radical application of the Mosaic rite of circumcision.*

Dr. J. Lewis Smith, the president of the Section, believed in the evil results of the reflex irritation due to abnormality of the prepuce. In many instances the causative relation of the preputial disease to the symptoms which it produces is not so apparent as it may be in others, but after correct treatment of the prepuce they disappear.

There was one result of phimosis which, he observed, neither Professor Sayre nor those who contributed to his paper noticed. The expulsive efforts accompanying urination sometimes cause prolapsus of the rectum, and frequently produce inguinal hernia. In a lecture before the Harveian Society (*British Medical Journal*, February 28, 1880), Edmund Owen, Surgeon to St. Mary's Hospital and to the Hospital for Sick Children, says:

> *Perhaps the commonest cause of hernia in childhood is a small preputial or urethral orifice, and next to that I would put the smegma-hiding or adherent prepuce.*

Arthur Kemp (London *Lancet*, July 27, 1878), Senior House-Surgeon to the Children's Hospital, says:

> *Phimosis is a common occurrence, and numerous ill effects can undoubtedly be attributed to it;*

and he alludes to the observation of Mr. Bryant, as published in his book on the *Surgical Diseases of Children*:

> *In fifty consecutive cases of congenital phimosis, thirty-one had hernia, five had double inguinal hernia, and many had umbilical hernia besides. In no one was the hernia congenital, its earliest occurrence being at three weeks. Circumcision was performed in these cases, and all were*

much benefited.[104]

---

[104] In looking over the literature of reflex neuroses and more direct injurious results, I find that George Macilwain, in a work *on Surgical Observations on the More Important Diseases of the Mucous Canals of the Body*, published in London in 1830, calls special attention to the case of a man aged thirty-eight, admitted to the Finsbury Dispensary, and who was in the care of Mr. Hancock. The patient was suffering from excruciating pain in different joints, the pain being so great that he was confined to his bed and unable to stand on his feet. He was unable to rest at nights, and neither rheumatic nor any other apparently suitable treatment was of any service. Rigors were soon added to his other troubles, and during their continuance the pain in his joints was greatly aggravated. He was referred to Mr. Macilwain for treatment, who promptly relieved him by the removal of a urethral stricture, which had quietly been the cause of all the disturbance. It is particularly interesting that even at that early day the reflex neuroses and complications that may arise from the irritability of the genito-urinary organs were so well understood. How well Dr. Macilwain appreciated the nicety of these relations can be seen from his remarks in connection with the above case, in which he says: "It may be observed that the severity of the symptoms is not always commensurate either with the duration of the disease or the degree of stricture, and that, although the progressive development of them varies considerably in rapidity, in different individuals, it is, nevertheless, in the latter stages, always more rapid." Macilwain also graphically describes the insidious approach of these genito-urinary troubles. In speaking of stricture he says: "Although minute inquiry generally informs us that the stricture has been of some standing, and in some instances has existed for years, yet it may happen that it is only a few months or a year since the patient's attention

has been directed to the disease. This is very intelligible; for, in conformity with what we observe in other parts of the body, the bladder has a power of accommodating itself to a change of circumstances. Its strength, for a long time, may increase so correctly in proportion to the increase of the obstacle which opposes the ejection of its contents that a very considerable period elapses before the difficulty in making water becomes cognizable to the patient, or it occasions an annoyance so trifling as scarcely to excite his attention. This increase of strength in the bladder frequently renders the formation of stricture so insidious that the urethra at the affected part is very narrow before the individual is aware of the existence of any contraction whatever; the bladder, however, at length becomes unable to empty itself, and the abdominal muscles and diaphragm powerfully act as coadjutors, so that each effort to make water is accompanied by a straining which is very distressing, and the complete evacuation of the bladder is often not accomplished even by these combined forces. The straining which accompanies stricture, and which seems necessary to evacuate the bladder, although it be occasionally exceedingly annoying to the patient at the time, is more important with reference to the results which are its consequence. I am firmly of opinion that there are a great number of patients laboring under hernia which has been produced by no other cause. I must confess that I had seen a great number of instances of stricture in ruptured patients before I drew any inference from the observation of their co-existence." The foregoing observations of Macilwain, made in 1830, are here reproduced for their clearness of expression and explanation, as well as to show what injuries can be produced on the young child afflicted with phimosis. We are, as surgeons, familiar with the anatomical and pathological changes there are undergone by the bladder and its lining membrane, as well as in the ureters and kidneys, in many cases of stricture, as well as of the great amount of prostatic irritability and enlargement that is due to the same cause. How similarly these results can be and are actually produced by phimosis is undeniably expressed by the post-mortem appearances in the poor infant described by Golding Bird to the London Medical Society, and mentioned in the London *Lancet* of May 16, 1846. The bladder and ureter were like those of a man who had long suffered from stricture. From the remarks of Dr. J. Lewis Smith, that phimosis may be productive of inguinal hernia and prolapsus of the rectum, and the observations of Edmund Owens and Arthur Kemp, both high authorities on children's diseases, being both connected with children's hospitals, as well as the remarks of Mr. Bryant in his "Surgical Diseases of Children," who all concur in looking upon phimosis as a great factor in hernia, Bryant having observed thirty-one in fifty consecutive cases of phimosis, we are certainly warranted in assuming that phimosis is not only a mere local timely inconvenience that will disappear with the approach of puberty, but a condition which, in the more easily affected organism of the child—lacking, as it does, that resistance that comes with our prime—is productive of serious harm; as even the first few years of life, even a few months of infant life, with a phimosis, are sufficient to so change the structures of parts that the poor child will grow into a man with an impaired kidney or sacculated ureter. The strain required to induce a prolapsus of the bowel or a rupture into the inguinal canal is exerted as much on the bladder, ureter, and kidney as on the other localities. Physicians who have taken the pains to observe must have noticed, more than once, how the child afflicted with a phimosis has not only at times to wait for the stream of urine to appear, there seemingly being some obstruction to its starting, but how often such a case is afflicted with a stammering, halting urination. A child thus

During the session of the Ninth International Congress, where the above paper was read and remarks made, which appear in the third volume of its *Transactions*, another paper was also presented by Dr. Saint-Germain, of Paris. The Doctor fully recognized the dangers from a narrow or adherent prepuce, but did not think that more than one case in three hundred really required circumcision; he believed in dilatation, as employed by Nelaton, with the exception that, whereas Nelaton employs three branches to his dilator, Saint-Germain preferred only a two-branch dilator.

Dr. Lewis, the president of the Section, related a number of cases where the use of uncleanly instruments had resulted disastrously. But, for that matter, the same objection can be offered against dilatation, as a filthy instrument is as liable to infect

---

started out into life, with a defective kidney or kidneys, is sadly handicapped in his usefulness, comfort, or in properly competing in the race of life. No parent would for a moment think of starting his son in life by giving him a business that is heavily mortgaged at the start, but many a parent unconsciously launches the unsuspecting child into a life of such ill health—resulting from a simple narrow prepuce—beside which a heavy mortgage or a heavy yearly tribute would be but a mere trifle. I have seen such men, who in after life, broken-down and perfectly physical wrecks, would gladly have given all their wealth and been willing to have some genii set them down in the middle of the Sahara, shirtless and pennyless, provided they had their health. To say nothing of the trifling loss of the prepuce, these parties would gladly have had a foot or a leg go with the prepuce if necessary, and have their health.

the patient as a knife.

There is no earthly excuse why a knife that has been used on a case of diphtheritic croup should be used some hours afterward to circumcise a child. As to the operation of dilatation practiced by Dr. Holgate, it can really be said to answer the *immediate* demands, but how far its utility is efficient as to *permanent* results Dr. Holgate has not given the profession any information.[105]

One of the most interesting and instructive papers that it was ever the fortune of the writer to listen to, touching on the subject of reflex nervous diseases or neuroses due to preputial adhesions, was one prepared by Dr. M. F. Price, of Colton, California, and read at the semi-annual meeting of the Southern California Medical Society, at its Pasadena meeting in December, 1889.

In the course of the paper he gives a considerable

---

[105] I have often performed dilatation where, for some reason, either the timidity of the parents or the health of the child seemed to contraindicate any more radical procedure. It is customary to advise mothers or the nurses to retract the skin daily, but even after a good dilatation I have found as sudden a recontraction, and even in the majority of cases, where daily drawing back the skin might have been racticable, the cries and struggles of the child are a positive prohibition to these instructions being carried out; it is not once in ten times that it can be carried out. I have seen two very annoying cases of paraphimosis resulting from this procedure, the struggles of the child having prevented the return of the prepuce to its proper place, and the violent crying and sobbing of the child having assisted to congest the organ.

number of examples, of which some extracts are herewith given: One case was a boy aged seven, who for two years had had frequent attacks of palpitation of the heart; when seen by Dr. Price the little heart was laboring hard, beating at a furious rate (far beyond counting), with a loud blowing or splashing sound, and the pulse at the wrist a mere flutter. The breath was inspired in a series of jerks, the face flushed and somewhat swollen. The chest-wall was visibly moved at every thump of the heart.

The doctor attended the child for a month without the little patient making any appreciable improvement. Some time during this period of observation the father happened to mention that the boy sometimes complained of his penis hurting him at the time of an erection. This led the doctor to examine the parts, when he found a long prepuce, with a mucous membrane adherent to the glans, about a line beyond the corona, the whole circumference of the organ.

With the use of cocaine and a blunt instrument the adhesions were removed, with an immediate amelioration of all the reflex symptoms. The very next paroxysm was lighter and less exhausting; the improvement was continuous. The child soon went to school and had no further trouble; but, in the doctor's opinion, the two years' hard struggle have not been without its evil results on the constitution and organism of the child.

The next case was born November 2, 1888; a large, healthy boy at birth. By June of the following year the child was afflicted with what the mother called "jerky spells;" up to this time the boy seemed listless, did not care to sit up, and seemed from some cause to be in more or less pain, with his eyes turned to the left.

The parents dreaded that the child, their only one, would turn out idiotic. The spasmodic spells alluded to were of a tetanic nature, the body being thrown backward; his head and eyes continued to be turned to the left, and nothing could attract the child's attention. The boy cried night and day, but he was in good flesh, had all the teeth he should have, bowels were regular, and the appetite good.

Whatever the doctor did in the medical way seemed to be of no avail. One day, however, he thought of examining the prepuce, thinking, perhaps, that it might be contracted and that the convulsive movements might be reflexes from the parts. On examination the prepuce was found elongated and distended, with a very minute opening; this was dilated with difficulty, when the inner fold was found adhering almost the whole extent of the glans; the dilatation and breaking down of these adhesions was slowly persevered in, until sufficient dilatation was obtained and the glans was freed.

From the very first operation the convulsions commenced to diminish, both in force and frequency, and a constant and rapid improvement of the child took place. Six months afterward the boy was perfectly normal, stood by himself, played with play-things, and was an interested member of the family circle.

Case No. 3 was a repetition of Case No. 2, except that, with the experience of the latter case, the doctor wasted no time with medication, but proceeded at once to examine the prepuce, which was found to be very long, and with a pin-hole opening. The dilatation of this and the breaking up of the adhesions gave immediate relief.

During the course of the paper he quoted the case related by Brown-Séquard, and recorded in the New York *Medical Record*, vol. xxxiv, p. 314, where he

> ...*related a very interesting case that presented all the rational signs of advanced cerebral disease, a case that he considered quite hopeless, that was relieved by an operation for phimosis and the treatment of an inflammatory condition of the glans penis.*

To use Brown-Séquard's own words,

> *So rapid was the recovery that within six weeks from the day of the operation he presented himself at my office perfectly well in every respect.*

In the early part of this book, in speaking of female circumcision, it was mentioned that when the medical part of the volume should be reached some medical reasons for its necessity would be given. Dr. Price, in his paper, gives some information on this subject, which is of the greatest interest. In the course of the paper he says as follows:

> *Nor do I think these reflex neuroses from adherent prepuce wholly confined to the male sex. The preputium-clitoridis may be adherent and produce in the female similar reflexes.*

During the session of the American Medical Association, held in Chicago in 1874, I think, I attended one afternoon a clinical lecture by Dr. Sayre. A little girl, fourteen years of age, but about the size of a seven-year-old child, was brought in, who had never walked nor spoken, but with quite an intelligent countenance, who was in constant motion, and who presented very many nervous symptoms.

Dr. Sayre examined her, and found the prepuce adherent the whole extent of the clitoris. He gave it as his opinion that here was the primary and sole cause of the symptoms, and that appropriate treatment shortly after birth would have prevented all the serious consequences so painfully apparent, and which was then too late to remedy.

I once had occasion to pass a catheter into the bladder of a lady who presented an innumerable train of nervous symptoms, often bordering on insanity, but was unable to do so without exposing the parts. Although the meatus could be distinctly felt, the catheter would not enter. On exposure to view, an opening was seen in the clitoris, which was firmly bound down by preputial adhesions near the extremity of the organ. Entering the catheter at this point, it readily passed through the clitoris, then down through a passage under the mucous membrane to the natural site of the meatus, on into the urethra, and through into the bladder. In the light of recent experience,

my opinion now is, that here was the cause
of all the nervous symptoms in this case.

The relative disposition in regard to the irritability of the external sexual organs as existing in the female, when contrasted with the male, is, for some reason, not sufficiently considered or understood.

The idea of masturbation or of irritation from the genitals ending in reflex neuroses is always, as a rule, associated with the male, and that it has not been more associated with the female has deprived her of the same benefit that the prosecution of the study in this regard has been to the male sex.

Masturbation among the feeble-minded, which is so common, must, of necessity, have for its determining cause a foundation of morbid irritability of the sexual organs. This is well known to be so among the males, whose hands seem instinctively to be drawn to those parts. Dr. C. F. Taylor, of New York, in an article on the *Effect of Imperfect Hygiene of the Sexual Function,* published in the *American Journal of Obstetrics* for January, 1882, gives us an account of his investigations in this regard, with the following results:

In an asylum for the feeble-minded of both sexes, it was found that the habit was about equal in the two sexes, there being only this difference: that the females began to masturbate one or two years earlier than the males, and that the habit, once established, was found to be more persistent than in the males. It was, further,

351

ascertained that the habit came naturally, without the aid of precept or example to either sex.

It may well be a question as to whether the feeble-mindedness be not a reflex condition from this excessive morbid irritability of the sexual organs.

There is not much doubt but that, if one of the cases reported by Dr. Price had not been circumcised, the expressionless, listless infant would have grown, in time, into a masturbating, feeble-minded, idiotic creature, as many others, so situated, have done before it.

Now, would it have been logical to have laid the morbid irritability of its generative organs to its feeble-mindedness, when its feeble-mindedness was fully demonstrated to have been wholly dependent on the sexual irritation? From these premises we might take another step forward, and ask whether, under a proper hygienic prophylaxis—which would involve a thorough inspection of the genitals of *all* children reported to be either physically or mentally deficient—such a course would not greatly diminish the number of paralytics, feeble-minded, and generally deficient of both sexes?

If the results in private practice are any criterion, it is safe to assert that a strict adherence to the Mosaic law for the males and to some of the African customs for the females would most assuredly relieve all these cases that might come under the caption of results of reflex neuroses. Twenty years ago this subject was, to the body of the profession, a *terra incognita* in regard to the male, and, as the female is similarly subject to the same morbid influence, it is to be hoped that in the present decade she will receive the same attention which the profession is now beginning to pay to the male sex.[106]

In the foregoing parts of this chapter, examples of reflex neuroses have been given to show the different effects that genital irritation will produce. The cases given were chosen for the diversity of variety of symptoms, and as cases representing the affection, without any other complication.

Many more could have been added, but they are unnecessary. In the writer's practice there has been a number of cases in the adult that have exemplified that this form of ailment is by no means restricted to children, as has been shown in the case reported by Dr. Mott to Dr. Sayre, in regard to the middle-aged man with a string about his penis.

One of these cases was that of a young man, six feet in stature, broad-shouldered, and well built. He applied for relief for a dyspepsia that affected his stomach and also his heart. The man had an apparently feeble and irritable heart; cold, clammy

---

[106] It may well be a question, considering the well-established fact that nervous injuries and affections are easily transmissible and become hereditary, how much feeble-mindedness is due to an heredity originally induced in either parent through reflex neuroses from the genital organs. The Jews have a very small percentage of feeble-minded; it is true that they have not any inebriates to assist in their manufacture, but still the absence of these well-pronounced cases of reflex neuroses among the race must be largely ascribed to their practice of circumcision, as that operation cures the gentiles so afflicted.

skin; disturbed digestion, and uneasy sleep; was constipated and flatulent. No treatment seemed to make any impression upon his case. At last he began to emaciate and look haggard. His mind was also becoming visibly weaker, was attacked by dizziness, and on several occasions he fell in a fit.

With this condition he at last began to have frequent nocturnal emissions. On account of the latter his genital organs were examined, and the penis was found smaller than the average, with a long and narrow prepuce. The glans could easily be uncovered, but the tightness of the prepuce and its unyielding qualities made paraphimosis a possibility; so that the young man, having once or twice had considerable difficulty in returning the prepuce to its place, never attempted its retraction again.

There were no adhesions, but the inner fold of the prepuce had been thickened by balanitis. Seeing the need of circumcision *for the local benefit*, the operation was suggested with a view of relieving the pressure on the glans, which was looked upon as the probable cause, in his broken-down condition, of the advent of the nocturnal emissions. He gladly submitted, and, to the surprise of both physician and patient, *all* his troubles disappeared, and he at once became a changed man.

So impressed was he with the result, that, on his return to his home, he examined his younger brother, and, finding him with a like long, narrow prepuce, he immediately brought him in and had him circumcised, as a prophylactic against his being subjected to the risk of lost health as he himself had suffered.

Another case, a man of forty-five, also a farmer,

was afflicted with dyspepsia, palpitation of the heart, general debility, constipation, constant headache, etc. He could not cut up an armful of wood without bringing on palpitations and gaseous eructations, or being upset for the day; and after having connection with his wife he generally had a terrific headache, lasting for two or three days; [107] he could stand no protracted mental effort, even such as is required to make an addition of a long line of figures, or the least business worry, without the supervening headache.

All treatment against these conditions was useless; the colon was kept empty, the diet was changed; pepsin and bismuth, tonics, frictions, Turkish baths, and all hygienic observances and moral treatment were all of no avail.

One day, on consulting the writer, he complained of a pruritus at the head of the penis. On examination it was found that he had a narrow, long prepuce, a congenitally-contracted meatus, and was then suffering with a slight balanitis. He was very careful to keep the parts clean, but, he informed me, that in spite of all precautions, these attacks would come on. The mucous covering of the inner fold of the prepuce and glans was so irritable that connection often brought it about.

The glans was small and elongated, with the

---

[107] I have seen precisely similar conditions resulting from a sphincterismus being relieved by anal dilatation. I had one such case who had fallen into the hands of a quack, who made him believe that he was being affected with incipient softening of the brain; systematic dilatation or a rupture of the sphincter *à la* Van Buren is the appropriate remedy.

meatus red, and with lips oedematous and congested. To free him from this tormenter, circumcision was advised. The party could not, however, remain away from home for the time required for the operation; so that a compromise operation was performed—one that would not keep him from business, and, at the same time, relieve the contracting pressure on the glans. This was by Clouquet's operation and bandaging back the prepuce over the penis, back of the corona—an operation that, in my hands, has often filled all the desired purpose. The meatus was also incised. After the operation *all* of his troubles disappeared, as they had done in the preceding case, and he was soon a hearty and well man, able to chop wood, attend to business, and, in case of need, do family duty for a Turkish harem without recurrence of his old tormenting, dyspeptic palpitation or sick-headache.

The writer has resorted to circumcision in many cases to improve the temper and disposition of children, with the best of results, and in one case, in association with another physician, performed the operation on a lunatic, whose lunacy ran to women and girls, with whom he would fall desperately in love, without any encouragement or provocation, or even acquaintance; finally reaching spells of such incoherence of action and speech that confinement would be required.

The peculiarity of his hallucinations called attention to the genital organs. This man had never masturbated, and was, when well, a compactly-built, active, and intelligent man. By occupation he was a contractor, and a man of more than usual executive ability besides.

On examination it was found that he was a subject of congenital phimosis, never having been able to uncover the glans. He had been in the habit of washing out the preputial cavity by the aid of a flat-nozzled syringe. The prepuce was long, but not thick; nevertheless, it was inelastic and very firm. The examination seemed to have a good mental effect upon the man, as it made him quite rational for the moment. He entered into the idea that this condition had some connection with his derangement very intelligently, even suggesting many symptoms and attacks that he had suffered from childhood up as probably gradual-stepping processes through which his present condition had been reached. He cheerfully submitted to a thorough circumcision, which had the effect of ameliorating his condition. He was subsequently sent to an asylum, where, after a short time, he was discharged well. Some years afterward, conscious of feeling a return of the mental derangement, he voluntarily applied for admission to the same institution and remained until better.

This case is very instructive. The patient readily connected his mental trouble, by a retrospective view through a series of gradually-increasing troubles, that originated in the preputial condition, to the phimosed condition of that appendage, and he was certain that this prepuce had been at the bottom of all the physical and mental trouble he had experienced.

The reflex nervous train of affections had undoubtedly produced some localized lesion in the brain-structure. The natural sound, healthy organism of that organ, and the bright, active nature of his mind, however, prevented a total wreckage of the mental faculties. It is safe to assume that, had he had the ordinary listless, unresisting mind, disposed to brood, and easily cast down, he would, from the first derangement, have become a hopeless and demented lunatic.

The circumcision could not undo all the mischief that had been accomplished, some of which had certainly left a permanent taint, but the mildness of his future attacks and the better exercise of his volition were the undoubted results of the operation.

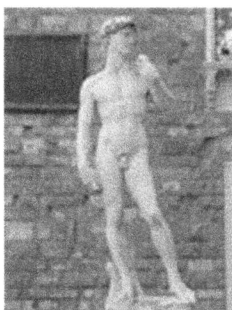

CHAPTER XXIV—DYSURIA, ENURESIS, AND RETENTION OF URINE

Any dissertation on circumcision and its many uses, either prophylactic or curative, would be incomplete without a reference to enuresis; another reason for making a somewhat full reference to the subject would be the undecided position that this morbid condition seems to occupy in medical literature, as well as the meagre and unsatisfactory treatment it has received by the majority of those who have mentioned it.

It is anomalous, to say the least, to find, in general or special literature, enuresis mentioned as a diseased condition peculiar from babyhood to puberty; to find it fully described and to have it stated that it is a widely-prevalent distemper, affecting both sexes alike; to know that it is an annoying, intractable, persistent condition, wearing to the child in every sense, subjecting it to a demoralizing mortification as well as to unmerited scoldings, humiliations, and punishments, and that its habit, in badly-ventilated

359

quarters, will breed other diseases,[108] as well as that its continued action tends to the development of onanism, with its long and widely-ramifying trains of physical and social ills; and to find works especially devoted to children's diseases silent on the subject.

Knowing all these things, and also that Ultzmann, Lallemand, and others who have treated this affection, mention it as a children's disease, it is unaccountable to reason out why most of our textbooks and treatises on children's diseases should be so remarkably and unreasonably silent. It certainly cannot be laid to its lacking in study material, as the author of *Quain's Dictionary of Medicine* says:

> *It is one relative to which much might be written without exhausting the subject, the*

---

[108] In the first volume of the American and English Encyclopedia of Law there is an interesting account of a young child (who had been bound out by the parish officials) who murdered his little bed-fellow and, on trial and conviction, was sentenced to be hanged, but who was reprieved by royal favor on account of his tender years, the sentence being changed to imprisonment for life. The little fellow was only eight years of age. On the trial the boy said he was driven to commit the crime because the other child soiled the bed. The two children being both paupers, it may well be imagined that their bedding was none of the cleanest at the best, or that their bed-room had the best of ventilation. As at the time the murder was committed English paupers were not treated in the most humane manner, it is not surprising that a nervous, sensitive child would, under such a combination of circumstances, be converted into an insane murderer.

pathology of which has wide and manifold relations.... There appears to be something analogous between this condition and that which determines in after life the seminal emissions under similar circumstances.

Our American works are notably deficient in this regard; Although Stewart, of New York, in his *Diseases of Children*, published over fifty years ago, devotes a chapter to dysuria and one to retention of urine, treating the subject quite fully, even down to the description of preputial calculi; he, however, failed to notice that the irritation of preputial constriction or adhesions will produce both conditions, and, following many of the authors of the time, as has been done since, he adopted the urino-digestion theory of acid and irritating urine, due to faulty digestion, of Prout and Magendie, who looked to regulating the digestion of the child, or the mother who nursed it, as the only method of cure; the lithic-acid diathesis being, in their opinion, the main thing to be guarded from.

Other works that mention these conditions are equally on the wide sea of speculation, as they all, more or less, look upon the treatment that they advise as indefinite and unsatisfactory, showing an equal want of sound anchorage-grounds for their etiological reasonings.

Dillnberger, of Vienna, in his handbook of children's diseases, mentions enuresis, but has nothing better to offer for its relief than that advised by Bednar, who followed a systematically-timed period of awakening, gradually lengthened out, from the time of putting the child to bed.

Peter Charles Remondino

In addition, he advises internal medication, and, like Ultzmann, he recognizes the possibility of a local cause in little girls, in whom he advises the local application of nitrate of silver. Edward Ellis mentions dysuria, and a long prepuce is noticed among its numerous causes. The works that give the subject the most intelligent treatment (the word "intelligent" is here used advisedly, and is in reference to the results obtained) are those of West, of London, and Henoch, of Berlin.

West, in his *Diseases of Children*, says:

> In the child, however, we sometimes find the symptoms produced by difficulty in making water owing to the length of the prepuce and the extreme narrowness of its orifice, which may even be scarcely large enough to admit the head of a pin. This congenital phimosis is, I may add, not an infrequent occasion of incontinence of urine in children, and is also an exciting cause of the habit of masturbation, owing to the discomfort and irritation which it constantly keeps up. In every case, therefore, where any difficulty attends the passing or the retention of the urine, or where the practice of masturbation is suspected, the penis ought to be examined, and circumcision performed if the preputial opening is too small. This little operation, too, ought never to be delayed, since, if put off, adhesions are very likely to form between the glans and the foreskin, which render the

necessary surgical proceeding less easy and more severe.

In the *Lectures on Diseases of Children*, Henoch, of Berlin, says:

> *I need scarcely add that an examination of the external genitals should never be omitted in any case of dysuria during childhood. You will not infrequently discover a phimosis which interferes more or less with the discharge of urine and retains portions of the latter behind the foreskin, where it may decompose and give rise to an inflammatory condition of the prepuce, with painful dysuria.... This is also true of the occasional adhesion of the labia minora in little girls, like the similar adhesion of the foreskin in boys. It is almost constant in the first period of life, but sometimes persists to the end of the first year; can usually be torn by the handle of the scalpel, and rarely requires an incision. In a few cases this adhesion appeared to me to be the cause of the dysuria, which disappeared after the separation of the labia from one another.*

Henoch, however, does not seem to have grasped the full relation that the natural phimosis of young children bears to dysuria, as he here follows the prevailing opinion, that where by dint, push, hauling, and hard work the prepuce can be pushed back phimosis does not exist, as well as the general apathy to the fact that a prepuce can exert a very injurious influence by its pressure, even when not adherent and very retractable; such a prepuce is often attended by balanitis and posthitis, with an accompanying difficult, frequent, and painful urination.

In a case which will be related farther on, in the discussion of the systemic effects of a long, contracted prepuce, as it induces diseased action by continuity of tissues, there is an account of a death of a two-year-old child which we can assume to have had its original starting-point in a condition of phimosis. Henoch, however, rather attributes the death in that case to what may well be considered the result of a cause, leaving the original cause more to appear as a final accessory condition.

My reasons for this view of the subject are simply owing to the fact that I do not believe that a child can long be afflicted with the *ischuria phimosica* of Sauvages without having the urinary organs beyond more or less seriously affected from the mere retention alone, irrespective of any reflex irritation from the pressure on the glans or of any from the irritation of the peripheral nerves; the dilatation of the adjacent cavities or channels and the deposit of calcareous matter being facilitated by the retention of urine and its naturally altered condition owing to that retention.

So that dysuria in young children, beginning in a slightly phimosed condition, or in the irritability of the glans and meatus, due to its preputial covering, it is safe to assume, may produce a train of symptoms ending in permanently-injured health, or even death.

The irritating urine of a slight access of fever may,

by its passage over the irritable mucous lining of the prepuce, be the initial starting-point of a serious or fatally-ending disease. In all of these, it must be admitted, the presence of the prepuce is either actively or passively the cause of the most serious disease processes that may follow.

Ultzmann, of Vienna, in his work on the *Neuroses of the Genito-Urinary Organs*, gives the subject of enuresis considerable attention. It is not a work on diseases of children, but it, nevertheless, goes into the subject as if it were, and furnishes the profession with considerable information. He defines enuresis to be the passage of urine of a normal quality in a child who, with the exception of this involuntary urination, is healthy.

In the first periods of life, a slight vesical or intestinal expulsive effort is sufficient to overcome the guarding sphincter muscles at their outlet; the child first obtains a voluntary control of the rectal sphincter; and, generally, with the second year it gains control of the vesical.

Those who pass their second year without obtaining this control, but in whom the organs and urine are normal, may be said to be afflicted with enuresis. He divides enuresis into three varieties; that involuntary urination which takes place at night during sleep he terms the *nocturnal*; that which takes place while climbing, laughing, coughing, or in the course of any violent muscular exercise is the *diurnal*; and that wherein the involuntary evacuation takes place day and night alike he terms as the *continued*.

This last is again subdivided into the continuous and periodical. As a cause, he cites anæmia, scrofula, rachitis; but adds that physical debility is not necessary for its presence, as well-developed, vigorous, puffy children are as liable to be affected as thin and scrawny ones; while not all scrofulous or rachitic children are so affected, only a small portion being enuretic.

Sex has no influence on the liability that tends to being attacked, the proportion between the sexes being about equal. As to age, he finds the greatest proportion to be between three and ten years, but he has often treated those of either sex even at the age of fourteen and up to seventeen years. It is absolutely necessary to examine the external genitals and the urine of those affected by this disease, as phlegmasiæ of the vagina, of the vestibule or urethra in girls, or the practice of onanism, or lithiasis, cystitis, or pyelitis may be the cause of the disease.

Girls are apt to be found affected with polypoid excrescences at the meatus, which when removed will cause the enuresis to disappear.

From the above it will be observed that Ultzmann has paid much attention to these neuroses; but it will also be remarked that neither the balanitis, collection of infantile smegma, preputial adhesions nor irritations are taken into any account as possible factors of either dysuria or enuresis; he has followed more or less an electrical form of treatment for genito-urinary neuroses, the rectal rheophore being one of his favorite modes of treating enuresis; in his etiologial views of these disturbances he has adhered more or less to the views of Trousseau, Bretonneau, and Dessault, who looked upon a debilitated or anomalous condition of the vesical neck as the cause of the majority of neuroses in that region.

It may be asked why these celebrated and observing physicians have neglected the preputial condition, if, as it is claimed, it is, in itself, so important and sure a factor of the derangements at the vesical neck?

To answer this, or to explain any marked discrepancy that may occur in medicine between minds equally as acute and observing, it is but necessary to observe that there is, in medicine, to a certain extent, a like rule of inheritance, education, with fashion or custom of habit of thought and practice, as we find in religion.

Canon Kingsley and Froude are equally as acute and discerning as the late Cardinal Newman, but that did not necessitate their following that prelate into the foremost ranks of the Catholic Church; and Pere Hyacynthe was equally as intelligent as Cardinal Newman, but that did not prevent him from leaving the fold into which the Cardinal had entered from out of the Reformed Church.

Some are born Catholics or Protestants, and are so with vehemence; others are born in these religions, but are only lukewarm in their doctrinal observance; while others reason and jump the traces in either direction. The followers of the destructive theories of Bronssais could not see the errors of their ways, and neither could they be made to see the merits of a less interfering form of medical practice.

Trousseau was himself at one time tainted with Bronssaisism, but, like Paul of Tarsus, he was made to see the error of his way, as he relates, through a case of gout that he nearly laid out in trying to lay out the disease antiphlogistically.

I do not assume that preputial irritation is at the bottom of *all* cases of dysuria or enuresis, any more than it would be rational to deny that cases of circumcision performed in some cases of diabetic enuresis have proved fatal as a result of the operative interference; but it is safe to assume that, in the great number of cases in whom some irritating conditions were found and removed, the enuresis or dysuria was due to such preputial irritation.

It is also logical to assume, with West and Henoch, that the organ should in all cases be examined, and its condition rendered as harmless as possible. That the condition of preputial irritation has not been fully recognized by all parties as a cause of enuresis does not do away with the fact that it does exist, any more than the refusal of the prelates and doctors of Salamanca to listen to Columbus did away with the fact of the existence of the American continents.

L. Ranney, in his *Lectures on Nervous Diseases,* pages 174, 175, speaks of enuresis in children as being a reflex cachexia,

> *excessive stimulation of the centripetal nerves connected with the so-called 'vesical centres' of the spinal cord,*

—a condition which may be produced by either worms in the intestines or by preputial irritation. Ranney advises a careful exploration of the urethra and rectum in these cases, and the elimination of all local causes of the conditions.

Probably the most remarkable case of the

immediate continuous effects resulting from phimosis is the one recorded by Vidal, in the fifth volume of the third edition of his *Surgery*.

This was a young man with a congenital phimosis, having but a very small aperture; on an operation to relieve the phimosis there was a gush of water, but this only fell at the feet of the patient, without being ejected at any distance; the urethra was found to have undergone precisely the same dilatation back of this preputial orifice that it usually undergoes back of a stricture; the whole urethra from the meatus backward was found to have exceeded the calibre of that of the vesical neck; the bladder was greatly dilated.

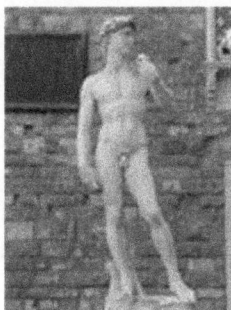

CHAPTER XXV—GENERAL SYSTEMIC DISEASES INDUCED BY THE PREPUCE

Aside from all the local affections or reflex neuroses, either mental or physical, that a prepuce may induce, there are an innumerable train of diseases that may originate in this one cause that at first sight would seem to have no connecting-link with any preputial condition.

It has already been suggested that the prepuce does not at all ages bear the same analogous relation to man. In childhood, especially during our earliest years, it is out of all proportion in size when compared to the rest of the organ, or to any use it may have placed to its credit.

Man does not, then, certainly need that refinement of nervous sensitiveness in the corona that is useful in after life in inducing the flow or ejaculation of the seminal fluid; neither is there at that age much of a corona to protect.

In middle life, or what might be called the procreative period of man, when the corona would seem to require all its excitability or sensitiveness, seems to be the very season in life when the glans is most apt to remain uncovered; so that nature and this hypothetical idea of the use of the prepuce are evidently at variance.

So we go through childhood with this long funnel-shaped appendage into manhood, when the increasing size of the body of the penis restores a sort of equilibrium between the size and bulk of the organ and its integumentary covering. At this period, as we have seen, although it does not, from the equilibrium restored, and the more or less use to which it is subjected, induce any great immediate or uncomplicated troubles, it nevertheless endangers the existence of the penis through the accidental course of some putrid or continued fever, or it subjects man to the manifold dangers of venereal or tubercular infections.

In advanced age, owing to the diminution in size of the organ, the prepuce resumes the proportionate bulky dimensions of childhood, and as the organ recedes and becomes more and more diminutive, the prepuce again, like in childhood, begins to tend to phimosis; the urine of the aged is also more irritating and prone to decomposition or putrefaction, and the constant state of moisture that the preputial canal of the aged is necessarily kept in, either by frequent urination or the incomplete emptying of the urethra that is peculiar to old age, and which results in more or less dribbling, is a powerful factor in inducing the many attacks of posthitis and balanitis, as well as those attacks of excoriation and eczema which are so annoying to the aged.

I have often seen such cases happening to men past fifty, who, being widowers, and never having had anything of the kind, as well as being in the most complete ignorance of the nature of the disease, have, from delicacy and fear that the disease might induce some suspicions as to their conduct in the minds of those whose good opinions they value above all else, gone on suffering untold miseries, especially if the urine were in the least diabetic.

One such case that fell under my observation not only produced such misery as to entail a loss of rest and of appetite, but even induced such a disturbance of assimilation and nutrition that the resulting hypochondriacal condition that developed from these enervating causes ran the patient into a low condition, ending in complete prostration of all vital powers and death, without the intervention of any other disease.

The subject was a timid, retiring man of about fifty-five years, and this was the first and only time that the prepuce had ever caused him any annoyance—a circumstance which greatly preyed upon his mind, as he could not disconnect it with the idea that it must be suspected as venereal, although he had always led a most continent life since the death of his wife.

This is, of course, an extreme case; but as it is a result beginning in a certain condition, be it an extreme, erratic, or infrequent occurrence, it is, nevertheless, an example of what may happen in advanced life, even where the prepuce has never before been a source of the least disturbance or annoyance. Persons who, with the increase of years, are also liable to an increase of adipose tissue, are more subject to this dwindling down of the penis and consequent elongation of the prepuce, with all the attendant annoyances, than thin or spare people.

In this irritation that the prepuce is liable to cause, we have not only to encounter the dangers that its thickenings or indurations may bring on in their train, in the shape of cancer, gangrene, or hypertrophies, but other and no less serious results are liable to follow a herpetic attack, or in consequence of an attack of balanitis or posthitis.

The dysuria attending any of these conditions may be the initial move for such a serious complication that life may be brought to a sudden end, even in infancy, to say nothing of the ease with which life is taken off in after years and in old age; with debilitated and imperfect kidney action, it takes very little to hustle us off from life's foot-bridge.

A case as occurring in Henoch's clinic, already mentioned or referred to in a previous chapter, shows what a simple phimosis is capable of inducing. In the history of the case the phimosis and the resulting retention in the preputial cavity no doubt were the causes of the calculus found there; and the succeeding calculi and abnormal condition of the urinary organs, we can safely assume, were a subsequent creation to that in the prepuce.

The case is taken from Henoch's *Lectures on Diseases of Children*, Wood Library edition, page 256, and is as follows:

A. L., aged two, admitted November 28, 1877. Quite well nourished, but pale. Complete retention of urine for two days;

373

slight redness and marked oedema of penis, scrotum, and perineum. The foreskin cannot be retracted, on account of phimosis. Abdomen distended, hard, and sensitive, the dilated bladder extending a few fingers' breadth above the symphysis. In order to introduce the catheter, it was first necessary to operate upon the phimosis, during which a calculus, which completely occluded the meatus, was removed. The catheter, when introduced into the bladder, removed a quantity of cloudy urine. The oedema, rapidly disappeared under applications of lead-wash, but on November 29th vomiting and diarrhoea occurred during the night, with rapid collapse; December 1st, death. Autopsy: In the bladder, a sulphur-yellow stone, as large as a hen's egg, completely filling the organ; similar calculi, from the size of a pea to that of a bean, in the pelvis of the left kidney; right kidney normal.

In the above case, the oedema of the penis, scrotum, and perineum was as much a result of the distension of the bladder by the retained urine interfering with the return circulation from the oedematous parts as the different appearances of diseased conditions were a result of the primary phimosis; yet this case, if seen during its early infancy, when probably the contraction of the preputial orifice was as yet not so well marked, would have been pronounced one in which it would be needless and barbarous to perform circumcision upon.

We would most assuredly have to wander aimlessly and unprofitably in the region of speculation to build up the etiology of the above-related case and reach the culmination there found, unless we accept the one that it was all, from first to last, the result of the phimosis.

Jonah, pitched overboard at sea to appease the tempest and swallowed by the whale, became convinced finally that he had better return to Nineveh to preach reform; while Pharaoh would not let the children of Israel depart even after Moses had so frightened him—as it is related in the rabbinical traditions compiled by the Rev. T. Baring-Gould, M.A.—that the royal bowels were completely relaxed at the sight of the snakes turned loose about the royal throne—a circumstance which nearly lost him his claim to divinity, which was based on the fact that his bowels moved only once a week, as in this case they not only moved out of time and in the most unkingly manner, so that the noble king hid underneath the throne, but before even Pharaoh could disengage himself from the royal robes, which event could hardly have raised him in the estimation of the gentlemen eunuchs of the bed-chamber.

Those who unwound the mummy of Pharaoh tell us that he had the appearance of a self-willed, despotic, but intelligent, old gentleman; but the above rabbinical relation, from Baring-Gould's *Legends of the Patriarchs and Prophets*, seems to have had no convincing effect on Pharaoh; so we must not be surprised if even a case like the one from Henoch's clinic would, with many, carry no conviction.

In the second volume of Otis on *Genito-Urinary*

Diseases, of the Birmingham edition, at page 380, there is an interesting account of a physician who, in youth, was troubled with an annoying prepuce, which, from frequent attacks of balanitis, had finally become more or less adherent to the glans penis; up to the age of nineteen he had been unable to completely uncover the glans. By six months of hard and persistent labor he had finally broken up these adhesions.

At the age of twenty-two he married, and he then ruptured the frenum, which bled profusely and left him sore for some days. Then for twenty-seven years he had no further trouble, but at the end of that time he began to experience what he believed were attacks of dumb ague, and the scrotum began to swell and felt sore on firm pressure. Heavy, aching pains then followed. This condition of things lasted for over five years, varied by the appearance of carbuncles on the nose and elsewhere, to relieve the monotony of the thing.

From this time on, abscesses began to form in the scrotum and into the integument of the penis, burrowing forward into the prepuce, which was much swollen and painful. A gangrenous opening effected itself in the dorsal surface, which relieved him somewhat. The patient was finally examined by Dr. Otis, who found a badly strictured urethra, the strictures beginning at the meatus, and at intervals extended down as far as two and three-fourths inches. The case had no venereal history, the patient never having had any disease or anything of the kind.

The strictures were plainly the result of the balano-posthitic attacks as much as they were the cause of the degeneration of the mucous membrane in the lower urethra, that allowed of the infiltration of urine into the tissues, which caused all the systemic disturbances, abscesses, misery, and agony of the patient, depriving him of comfort, sleep, or ability for labor, and which sent him here and there in search of health and relief.

It would seem really as if a prepuce was a dangerous appendage at any time, and life-insurance companies should class the wearer of a prepuce under the head of hazardous risks, for a circumcised laborer in a powder-mill or a circumcised brakeman or locomotive engineer runs actually less risk than an uncircumcised tailor or watchmaker.

They recognize the danger that lurks in a stricture, but what a prepuce can and does do, they entirely ignore. I have not had any opportunities for comparison, but it would be interesting to know, from the statistics of some of these companies, how much more the Hebrew is, as a premium-payer, of value to the company than his uncircumcised brother.

Were they to offer some inducement, in the shape of lower rates, to the circumcised, as they should do, they would not only benefit the companies by insuring a longer number of years, on which the insured would pay premiums, but they would be instrumental in decreasing the death-rate and extending longevity.

I have seen so many cases of stricture whose origin could be traced to balanitis that it can almost with confidence be assumed that, wherever there is a long prepuce with a red and inflamed meatus in a child, that unfortunate child will be a victim of fossal strictures when arrived to manhood, and that, moreover, he will be a surer victim to the reflex neuroses which so often accompany strictures, and which have been so ably described by Otis, than the victim of uncomplicated strictures acquired in the worship of Venus.

There is no end to the misery that these poor fellows have to suffer, besides the habitual hypochondriacal condition into which the accompanying physical depression, throws them; it unfits them for business, any undertaking, or even for social enjoyment or entertainment; they keep themselves and their families in continued hot water. These subjects are, also, more prone to gouty and rheumatic affections, asthma, and other neuroses.

Among the many cases of nervous disorders simulating other diseases that I have seen relieved were two Jewish lads with an imperfection of the meatus. They were two brothers, and from the history of the cases, and that given me by the mother of the lads in regard to the father, the malformation must have been hereditary and congenital. It consisted of a partial occlusion of the meatus by a false membrane, which divided the meatus in two, horizontally, but which was closed at the posterior end of the lower passage, which readily admitted a probe from the front as far as the occlusion, about a third of an inch to the rear. The restoration, or rather the making the anterior urethra and meatus to their normal condition, relieved both boys of asthma, under which they had labored for years.

The many cases simulating the general disturbances that accompany many kidney disorders, that are simply the result, in their primary causes, of preputial irritation and the disturbances to the kidney function due to the same cause, have long induced me to look upon the prepuce as a great and avoidable factor to some of the many forms of kidney diseases, prostatic enlargements, vesical diseases, and many other diseases of the urinary organs, which we know full well can result from strictures, as the latter need not always act in a purely mechanical mode to do its full extent of mischief.

One result of these preputial irritations not generally or particularly mentioned in any of our textbooks—a condition far-reaching as regards its own results, and more annoying and serious than it appears at first sight—usually begins with a reflex irritability of the anal sphincter muscle, or a rectal irritation of the same order, which in time produces such organic change that an hypertrophied and irritable, indurated, unyielding muscle is the result.

Agnew, of Philadelphia, describes the condition, but does not mention this frequent cause under the name of sphincterismus; once this is established, the train of resulting pathological or diseased conditions that may follow are without end.[109] This is no fancy

---

[109] The study of prematurely acquired impotence in the male is a most interesting one. I have frequently seen it result from the presence of anal or rectal irritation, from hæmorrhoids. I have seen cases who could not have erections, and in whom all sexual desire was extinct at a very early age, who have informed me that, although unable to have sexual intercourse because of the total absence of sexual desire, the flaccidity of the organ, and the want of sound physiological organic functional activity to suggest the thought, they had, nevertheless, frequently been the victims of nocturnal emissions before the total extinction of

the function. As a rule, much of this premature impotence—induced by either irritation of the genital organs or rectal or anal troubles—runs its unfortunate possessor through such a course of physical incidents as described by Hammond, as the wild Indians of the Southwest induce in the *mujerado*. At first the sound organ responds in a natural manner to any stimulus that may affect it, but soon a local satyriacal condition is set up, which, running a more or less rapid period of intense activity, soon leaves its victim completely, permanently, and hopelessly impotent, even as much so as if eunuchized in the most approved manner. Hammond's description of the manner in which these unfortunates are manufactured is an interesting addition to the facts contained in the natural history of man, and is as follows: "A *mujerado* is an essential person in the saturnalia, or orgies, in which these Indians, like the ancient Greeks, Egyptians, and other nations, indulge. He is the chief passive agent in the pederastic ceremonies which form so important a part in the performances. These take place in the spring of every year, and are conducted with the utmost secrecy, as regards the non-Indian part of the population. For the making of a *mujerado* one of the most virile men is selected, and the act of masturbation is performed upon him many times every day; at the same time he is made to ride almost continuously on horseback. The genital organs are thus brought, at first, into a state of extreme erethism, so that the motion of the horse is sufficient to produce a discharge of seminal fluid, while at the same time the pressure of the body on the animal's back—for the riding is done without a saddle—interferes with their proper nutrition. It eventually happens that, though an orgasm may be caused, emissions can no longer be effected, even upon the most intense degree of excitation. Finally, the accomplishment of an orgasm becomes impossible; in the meantime the penis and testicles begin to shrink, and in time reach their lowest plane of degradation.

But the most decided changes are at the same time going on, little by little, in the instincts and proclivities of the subject. He loses his taste for those sports and occupations in which he formerly indulged, his courage disappears, and he becomes timid to such an extent that, if he is a man occupying a prominent place in the council of the pueblo, he is at once relieved of all power and responsibility, and his influence is at an end. If he is married his wife and children pass from under his control— whether, however, through his wish or theirs, or by the orders of the council, I could not ascertain. They certainly become no more to him than other women and children of the pueblo." Hammond examined one of these men, who had, as he himself informed him, formerly possessed a large penis and testicles "grande como huevos,"—as large as eggs. The penis was in its flaccid state and about an inch and a half in length, with the glans about the size of a thimble, which it very much resembled in shape. The glandular structure of the testicles had disappeared; they were atrophied, little besides connective tissue remaining. He examined another *mujerado* in the pueblo of Acoma, who had been so made when at about the age of twenty-six. The penis was not more than an inch in length and about the diameter of the little finger, and of the testicles there was apparently nothing left but a little connective tissue. Both of these men had high-pitched voices. The last one examined was then thirty-six years of age. (Hammond: *Male Impotence.*) The foregoing detailed description shows an extreme degree of results produced by an equally extreme degree of intense and persistent irritation applied to the genital organs, purposely employed to obtain certain results. In the cases cited the irritation or excitation is directly applied, but it is safe to assume that reflex irritability from the anus or rectum, or from that of a stricture or of a prepuce, will in some cases produce a certain degree of excitation in the testicles that may result in their functional or organic derangement, in a degree proportionate to that of the amount of excitation from which they have suffered. That the testicles are very apt to suffer from the existence of a stricture is a well-known fact. I have myself worried over a case of stricture, in whom the attempted passage of a filiform bougie was always immediately followed by a severe attack of epididymitis, and who had always been afflicted with a tenderness and a tendency to inflammation of the testes. I have also noticed a much greater tendency to orchitis in the wearer of an irritating prepuce than where it was absent; so that the presence of a satyriacal tendency, no matter in what proportion of a degree it may be present, can safely be assumed to result in a corresponding degree of apathy, due to an actual physical degeneration of the parts. That these conditions, when present in any degree of permanency or persistence, will in the end induce early impotence, I have no reason to doubt. In this regard we must not overlook the fact that persons with phimosis, stricture, or other genital irritants and impediments, are more liable to be afflicted with hæmorrhoids, prolapsus ani, or other anal and rectal irritation, which retroactively assist in bringing about the condition under question. How much this may have to do with certain prolific peculiarities among the Jews may well be questioned; it is a well-known fact that in London the Jewish excess of male births has been as high as eighteen per cent., while among the Christian or Gentile population it is only six and one-half per cent.—a somewhat analogous condition of proportion being also observable in the United States. Here, it is accounted for, in a measure, by Dr. Billings, in the following words: "This comparatively large proportion of males among the Jews is probably due to the fact that the death-rate of their infants sketch, nor will the student of the pedigree and origin of diseases feel that the case is exaggerated or imaginative.

These are some of those cases that are always ailing, never well and really never sick, but who are, nevertheless, gradually breaking down and finally die of what is termed "a complication of diseases," before living out half their term of life.

How this happens is simple enough—the straining required to produce an evacuation is out of all proportion with the character of the discharge; such

---

is less for males, as compared with females, than it is among the average population." Children gotten during the prime of life of the parents are naturally more virile and have better stamina than those gotten before full maturity is reached. If the father is on the verge of impotency just about the time he is expected to beget his best offspring, that offspring cannot be expected to present an extra amount of vitality, virility, or physical stamina; hence, the prepuce can be brought in as directly tending—in no matter how small the degree it may be, but nevertheless a factor— to the physical degeneracy of the race, as well as it demonstrates the existence of some law for the production of the sexes which we do not as yet fully comprehend. Aside from the above considerations, there are those of the actual bar to the increase of population which the prepuce induces, either by primarily being the cause of impotence or by direct interference, as already mentioned, and the impotence that naturally results from the causes set forth in this note. The results of a prepuce are certainly such as must act like a moist, warm, and oily poultice to the irritability induced in the most confirmed Malthusian when contemplating the—to him—rapid and unwarranted increase of population.

patients often complain of being constipated when the evacuations are semi-fluid; this straining is followed by a dilatation and consequent loss of power of the rectum, which becomes pouched and its mucous membrane thickened; the whole intestinal tract sympathizes and digestion is interfered with, and the forcible expulsive efforts affect all the abdominal and thoracic organs in a more or less degree, laying the foundation for serious organic diseases.

Now, this condition, which may be said to be no more than one of obstinate constipation, is a far more reaching condition and a far more injurious state than can be imagined at a first glance. Constipation is not, as a rule, always accompanied by the indigestion, either stomachic or intestinal, that goes with this condition; the contents of the intestines in simple constipation may simply lack fluidity without undergoing putrefactive fermentation, but in this condition the undigested and retained intestinal contents do undergo that change, resulting in the generation of material whose re-absorption produces a toxic condition of the blood, from whence begins a series of serious organic changes in the blood, and from this in the organs.

To the practical physician these changes are evident and their cause just as plain, and it is just here where the laity lack the proper education, and where they should understand that the intelligent physician generalizes the disease and only individualizes the patient; and it is this ignorance on the part of the laity that gives to empiricism and quackery that advantage over them, as they look upon all disease as a distinct individual ailment, that should have an equally distinct and individual therapeutic agent to cope singly with.

The laity know very little of these things, and in their happy ignorance care still less for the finer definitions of or of the clinical importance of toxæmia, or the processes of abnormal conditions that lead up to such a state, or the results that may follow when that condition is once reached. To them, dyspepsia is an indigestion ascribable to the stomach, and a sick-headache is ascribed to something wrong about the stomach or liver.

The laity have never been called upon to answer the questioning of the late Prof. Robley Dunglison:

What do you mean, sir, by biliousness? Do you mean, sir, that the liver does not secrete or manufacture a sufficiency of bile, or not enough? Do you mean that the bile-material is left in the blood, or too much poured in? Do you mean that there is an excess in the alimentary canal, and a deficiency elsewhere? Please, sir, explain what you really mean by the term 'bilious!'

The Professor had a way about him that at least made one stop and seriously inquire, before adopting any random notion in regard to medicine.

It is to be regretted that, in the humdrum tread-mill work of many physicians, they even have to drop into the commonplace way of treating dyspepsias and such ailments without any further inquiry. A farmer knows better than to drive a dishing wheel, or with merely having a nail clinched in the loose shoe of a valuable horse; but he is fully satisfied to do so in a metaphorical sense, as regards his own constitution, and the mere hint from his physician that he had better lay up for repairs, or that there is something wrong about him that will require investigation, and that there is an ulterior cause to his feeling tired, headachy, or dyspeptic, or an allusion that there is something systemic, as a cause, to his momentary attacks of disordered vision or amaurosis, will generally make him look on the doctor with mistrust.

The merchant, banker, and mechanic are not up to Professor von Jaksch's ideas of toxæmia—that toxæmia may be exogenous or endogenous, or that the latter is further subdivided into three more varieties— and, what is worse, he cares still less.

The above three classes of humanity, when sick, simply would want to know if Professor von Jaksch was good on dyspepsia, the measles, or typhoid fever. They care very little that he divides endogenous or auto-toxæmia into that produced by the normal products of tissue-interchange, abnormally retained in the body, giving rise to uræmia, toxæmia from acute intestinal obstruction, etc., the above being the first division.

The second depends on the outcome of pathological processes, which change the normal course of assimilation of food and tissue-interchange; so that, instead of non-toxic, toxic matter is formed. The second group he names noso-toxicoses, which he subdivides into two principal divisions:

(a) The carbohydrates, fats, or albuminous matter, which may be decomposed abnormally and give rise to toxic products, *e.g.*, diabetic intoxication, coma carcinomatosum.

(*b*) A *contagium vivum* enters the body through the skin, or the respiratory or digestive tract, and develops toxic agents in the tissues on which it feeds, as in infectious diseases.

In the third group the toxic substance results from pathological non-toxic products, which again produce a toxic agent, only under certain conditions.

This group he calls auto-toxicoses, and includes in it poisonous substances, resulting from decomposition of the urine in the bladder, under certain pathological conditions, and giving rise to the condition called ammoniæmia. (*Medical News* of January 7, 1891; from *Wiener klinische Wochenschrift* of December 25, 1890.)

As observed above, unfortunately the patients know nothing, nor can they be made to understand these conditions, that are only reached through labyrinthic pathological processes, and, what is still worse, this way of looking at disease is incompatible with the idea of specific-disease treatment, which to them looks more practicable and quick, and which is also more to their liking. They cannot see any sense in such reasoning, which to them is something eminently impracticable; neither can they see a reasonable being in the doctor who practices on such, as they call them, *theories.*

The practical physician, however, sees in Professor von Jaksch's summary the turning-point of many a poor fellow's career—from one of comparative health into one of organic disintegration, decay, and dissolution—all the required processes starting visibly from the very smallest of beginnings; any obstruction in the urinary tract or intestinal canal being sufficient to start any of the conditions which end in toxæmia; and, from a careful observation running over several years, I do not think that I am assuming too much in saying that a balanitis is often the tiny match that lights the train that later explodes in an apoplectic attack or sudden heart-failure due to toxæmia; the organic and vascular systems being gradually undermined until, unannounced and unawares, the ground gives way and the final catastrophe occurs— unfortunately, an occurrence or ending looked upon as unavoidable by the friends of the victim.

They cannot see any danger; the idea that diseases have the road paved, not only for an easy entrance but an easy conquest, by the action of these toxic agents on the tissues, is something that they cannot grasp.

These blood changes or blood conditions are things too intricate, and the physician who understands them is, to them, a visionary and unpractical man. These conditions are, however, neither new nor unknown, and there is really no excuse for the ignorance exhibited in these matters by the general public, as it is through the blood that this mischief takes place. They can reason in their impotent way, that they should drench themselves with "blood tonics" and all manner of nauseous compounds to "purify" their blood, but the simple, scientific truth is something beyond their understanding, as well as something that they steel themselves against.

Sir Lionel Beale, in observing the immense importance he attaches to blood composition and blood change in diseases of various organs, truly remarks that

...blood change is the starting-point, and may be looked upon as the cause, of what follows...

the other factor being the "'tendency or inherent weakness or developmental defect of the organ which is the subject of attack;'" to which he adds that he feels convinced that, if only the blood could be kept right, thousands of serious cases of illness would not occur; while the persistence of a healthy state of the blood is the explanation of the fact that many get through a long life without a single attack of illness, although they may have several weak organs; and that an altered state of the blood, a departure from the normal physiological condition, often explains the first step in many forms of acute or chronic disease.

Sir Lionel has been a pioneer in the field of thought that looks for the cause of the disease, which, however remote it may be, should not be overlooked as a really primary affection. His extensive labor in the microscopic field has fully convinced him that many of the pathological changes in the different organs are due to what might be called some intercellular substance that is deposited from the blood. (Beale: *Urinary and Renal Disorders.*)

Toxic elements in the blood affect the kidneys in a greater or less degree, and there produce changes at first unnoticed—at least, as long as the kidney can perform its function—but the day arrives when, as described by Fothergill, blood depuration is imperfect, and we get many diseases which are distinctly uræmic in character, and ending in any of the so-called kidney diseases, Bright's disease being one of the most common.

As observed by Fothergill, however, the kidney is not the starting-point, the new departure only taking place when the structural change on the kidney has reached that point that it is no longer equal to its function—the "renal inadequacy" of Sir Andrew Clarke. (J. Milner Fothergill, in the *Satellite*, February, 1889.)

During the Bradshawe lecture, Dr. William Carter made the following remarks:

> *According to Bonchard, one-fifth of the total toxicity of normal urines is due to the poisonous products re-absorbed into the blood from the intestines, and resulting from putrefactive changes which the residue of the food undergoes there.*

In the course of the lecture, Dr. Carter fully explains that one of the benefits derived from milk diet in Bright's disease is the small residuum deficient in toxic properties, and lays great stress on the employment of intestinal disinfectants or antiseptics that exercise their influence throughout the whole tract, suggesting naphthalin as peculiarly efficacious, thereby cutting off one source of blood contamination at its source. Although these are recent developments in medicine, Bonchard mentions that in the practice of M. Tapret cases treated on this principle did well. (Braithwaite's *Retrospect*, January, 1889.)

Persons laboring under this toxic condition of the

blood, with a consequent deterioration in the texture and the physiological function of the vital organs, are of that class that easily succumb to injuries or serious sickness, and of that class to whom a surgical operation of even medium magnitude is equal to a death-warrant.

The above conditions are an almost constant attendant on that condition of the sphincter described by Agnew as sphincterismus, which also is productive of hæmorrhoids and fissure, and often of fistula. That sphincterismus is caused in many cases by preputial irritation is as evident as that the same affection, or hæmorrhoids or any other rectal or anal affection, will, in its turn, produce vesical and urethral reflex actions, and primarily functional and secondarily organic changes in those parts.

Besides, the great number of cases wherein the gradual and progressive march of each pathological event could be traced with accuracy has convinced me of the true cause of the difficulty being the result of reflex irritation.

Delafield, in his *Studies in Pathological Anatomy*, gives, as the first form of pneumonia, that from heart disease; in the days of Broussais this would have sounded absurd, but, to-day, some forms of heart disease are known to be the regular sequences of some particular form of kidney disease, just as some form of pneumonia attends an affected heart and that some forms of pneumonia degenerate into phthisis.

When the blood change is an established fact, it is only a question as to which is the weak organ, and the organism of the individual will decide whether it will be a simple sick-headache or the beginning of a pneumonia ending in phthisis.

I have purposely dwelt on this part of this subject, owing to the recent origin and publication of many of the views connected with it; also on account of the greater ease of making the subject plain by fully discussing each step of the process; and if the views of Sir Lionel will be recalled, that a toxic element in the blood is the starting-point, and that an irritable or weakened organ invites destruction—the induction of serious and fatal kidney disorder by the transmitted irritability and consequent injury to the kidney produced by preputial irritation in the first instance, and the supplemental blood-poisoning by intestinal absorption of septic matter, which soon brings about Sir Andrew Clarke's "inadequacy of kidney,"—all will be readily understood.

When this point is reached, a too hearty meal, exposure to variable weather, or a little extra care or anxiety, are sufficient, as determining causes, to bring life into danger.

As pointed out, many cases of Bright's disease or other renal difficulty have their origin in this distant but visible source, and, although malarial poisoning and a great number of other causes will produce the same particular organic changes and diseases, this condition must be admitted as one of the frequent causes.

The influence of the genito-urinary tract on the rest of the economy, and the importance of the sympathy it excites, or how quickly, by its being irritated, some apparently dormant pathological condition will be awakened to life and activity, is not sufficiently appreciated. As observed by Hutchinson, a patient who has once been the subject of intermittent fever is more prone, on catheterization, to have a urethral chill and fever than one who had never had the fever. (Hutchinson: *Pedigree of Diseases*.)

Ralfe observes, in his *Kidney Diseases*, that long-standing disease of the genito-urinary passages must be reckoned as among the chief etiological factors of chronic interstitial nephritis (page 227). The condition of the kidneys in cases of strictures of long standing is known not to be a reliable one, and any incentive to dysuria or to retention, no matter how slight, is apt to lead, eventually—and that even in very young subjects—to that toxic condition mentioned in a former part of this chapter as one of von Jaksch's subdivisions of toxæmia, the ammoniæmia of Frerichs; this condition being the fatal ending of the case of the two-year-old child mentioned by Henoch, who died after the relief of a retention due to phimosis and calculi resulting from the phimotic occlusion.

Having seen so many cases wherein the conditions described in this chapter were so apparently—whether from ammoniæmia due to infection, or toxæmia from the urinary tract, or uræmic toxæmia from the intestinal tract—all due to some preputial interference or irritation, I cannot help but feel that in these conditions—which, singularly, are not so prevalent with the Hebrews as with Christians—we have one factor in the cause of the shorter and more precarious vitality of the latter.

Morel, in his *Traité des Dégénérescences Phisiques*, ably discusses the degenerative and morbific influences and results of toxæmia, as well as he clearly defines their sources. The connection between toxæmia and mental affections has already been shown, and Prof. Hobart A. Hare, in his instructive and interesting prize essay on *La Pathogénie et la Thérapeutique de l'Épilepsie* (Bruxelles, 1890), mentions that convulsive disorders resulting from the presence of some toxic substance are of frequent occurrence.

How much this may enter as a partial factor into many of the cases of epilepsy which are classed in the order of "reflex" may well challenge our consideration. Hare lays great stress on the necessity of circumcision wherever there is an indication of preputial local irritation.

> *If practicable, circumcision should be performed; it is an operation with but small risk or danger, and easy of performance. In such circumstances it is always permissible to circumcise, were it for no other end than an acknowledged attempt to reach a cure.*

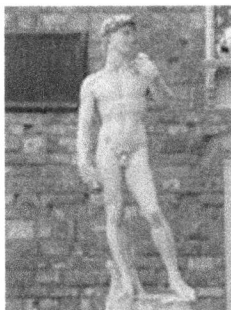

CHAPTER XXVI—SURGICAL OPERATIONS PERFORMED ON THE PREPUCE

In operative interference there is one point which should not be lost sight of, this being that the length and bulk of the prepuce in a great measure depends on the constriction at its orifice; if the orifice is small, the prepuce tight and inelastic, every erection, by putting the penis-integument on the stretch, adds to its bulk— nature naturally trying to make up the deficiency—the two points of resistance being where the glans pushes it ahead, having the constricting orifice for a hold or purchase, and the skin at the pubes, which is called upon to furnish the extra tissue for the time being needed during erection, which should be supplied by the prepuce—this being the only office which I have been able to assign to this otherwise useless but very mischievous appendage.

In cases where preputial irritation produces more or less priapism, the continued stretching of this integument causes a marked increase in its growth, which is mostly added forward. It was on this principle or its recognition, that Celsus devised his operations, and on which the persecuted Jews undertook to recover their glans by manufacturing a prepuce; and, although the trial was not reported as being very successful, I do not doubt but that, if the skin could have been drawn sufficiently over so as to constrict it anteriorly so as to give the glans a purchase, as in the case of phimosis with an inelastic prepuce, the operation could be more of a success; all that is required is the continued extension and the prepuce might be made to rival in length the labia majoræ of the females of some African tribes, or the pendulous buttocks of the Hottentot Venus.

I have employed the knowledge of this elasticity and source of supply of the penis-integument, on more than one occasion, in recovering the denuded organ with skin. A number of cases are on record where, owing to the want of that artistic and mechanical knowledge without which no surgeon is perfect, the operator has drawn forward the skin too tight in circumcising, after which, owing to the natural elasticity of the skin, the integument has retracted, leaving the penis like a skinned eel or sausage.

This accident is even liable to occur where the skin has not been tightly drawn, but where subsequent erections have torn through the sutures, and where the natural retraction of the skin has laid the organ bare for some distance. I have seen a number so recorded, but do not remember seeing any remedy suggested, it seemingly being accepted that the recovery must take place by gradual granulation—a necessarily very slow process, owing to the constant interference by—the always present in such cases—

unavoidable erections.

Several years ago I advised circumcision to a gentleman owing to a contracted condition of the muscles of one hip and thigh, which was threatening to render him a deformed cripple; he had a congenital phimosis and a very irritable glans penis.

The operation was performed in a proper manner by a surgical friend, but this friend, unfortunately, was a great believer in antiseptic and wet dressings. A few days after the operation he called upon me to ask me to go and see the patient, as they were both in a pickle, the patient being exceedingly angry, being in constant misery, and the penis so denuded by the giving way of the sutures—owing to the erections—that it looked to the patient as if he never could have a whole penis again, and the doctor saw no way out of the difficulty; the penis was, in reality, a dilapidated and sorrowful-looking appendage, and anything else but a thing of beauty or pride; it was raw, angry-looking, and bleeding at every move; the first wink of sleep was followed by an attempt at erection that raised the patient as effectually as an Indian would in scalping him; so that, taken altogether, the penis, anxious countenance, and the flexed position of the whole body to relieve the tension on the organ, the man looked about as battered, cast down, and sorrowful as Don Quixote did in the garret of the old Spanish inn, with his plastered ribs and demolished lantern-jaw.

Luckily, the patient was seen before the retracted portion of the penile integument had had a chance to condense and indurate. The bed was slopping wet with the drenchings of carbolized water that the penis had undergone, the man's clothing was necessarily damp, and the whole bedding and clothes were steamy—all of which greatly added to his discomfort and tendency to erections.

The man was washed, placed in a new, clean, and dry bed, and his clothing changed. The organ was then forced backward until the preputial frill or edge was approximated to the cut end of the penis-skin, where it was made fast by an uninterrupted suture around the whole of the circumference. A short catheter, about three inches in length—the catheter being as full size as the urethra would comfortably hold, and of the best and thickest of the red, stiff variety—was introduced into the urethra.

This protruded about half an inch beyond the meatus. A stiff, square piece of card-board was pierced and slipped over this, and then adhesive rubber straps were brought from the integument to this little platform, the first being from the median line of the scrotum, lifting the sac forward and upward. The pubes were shaved and the next four straps started from the root of the penis, each strap being split at the glans-end so as to encircle the protruding end of the catheter.

By these means the skin was brought back and firmly supported over the penis, toward the glans; and, in case of any erection, the act would only assist in drawing the covering farther over the penis as the pasteboard platform and adhesive straps formed the distal end of an artificial phimosis. The catheter allowed of free urination, and the scrotum was further held up in position by a flat suspensory bandage passed underneath the scrotum and fastened over the abdomen near each hip. The penis wound was then dressed with a very little benzoated oxide-of-zinc ointment passed between the adhesive straps; a bridge-support placed over the hips to support the bed-clothes, and all was finished, and full doses of bromide of sodium and chloral were ordered at bed-time.

When the dressings were removed, five days afterward, all was healed, the sutures removed, and the suspensory alone replaced. The patient had not been troubled with any more erections or annoyances of any kind. These are the points which often do more or less mischief: wet dressings are uncomfortable and favor erections, while the effect of the weight and action of the scrotum in drawing backward on the integument should not be overlooked; in addition, it should not be overlooked that we have it in our power to produce, so to speak, an artificial phimotic action, which has the same traction on the penis-integument that the natural phimosis induces.

The foregoing method, to be used in these cases, has proved very serviceable in my hands, and it is here given that it may assist others; as there is no need of waiting for granulations or of allowing the patient to undergo so much misery, which, besides the local injury, cannot help but affect the general health very injuriously.

The penis can stand any amount of forcing backward; it stands this in cancer or hypertrophy of the prepuce, or in the inflammatory thickenings that precede gangrene of the prepuce, in any extended degree; becoming, for the time being, more or less atrophied. As has been shown by Lisfranc, the penis can be made nearly to disappear into the pubes; so that we are not as helpless in these cases as our text-books would have us believe.

In infants, and in young children below the age of ten or twelve, the Jewish operation, as modified and done in accordance with the dictates of modern surgery, will be found the most expedient. By this method we avoid the need of any anæsthetic agents, which are more or less dangerous with children, as well as the need of sutures, which are painful of adjustment and very annoying to remove in those little fellows who dread new harm; there is also much less risk of hæmmorrhages, as the frenal artery is not wounded.

In children of a year or over, a very good result will be found often to follow Cloquet's operation, care being taken to carry the slitting well back, as well as care in taking it on one side of the frenum, so as to avoid any wound of that artery, the subsequent dressing being a small Maltese-cross bandage, pierced so as to admit the glans to pass through; the prepuce is retracted and the tails folded over each other and held there by a small strip of rubber adhesive plaster; a little vaselin prevents the soiling by urine underneath.

This last operation is short and very easy, is not painful, nor does it require much manipulation; it is only one quick cut on the grooved director and it is over; by the retraction of the prepuce, the longitudinal cut becomes a transverse one, making the prepuce wider and shorter at once; the glans soon develops and remains uncovered. As there is a very small wound to heal over, the repair is very prompt.

In adults with a very narrow, thin, not overlong prepuce, a very good result often follows a combination of the dorsal slit with the inferior slit alongside of the frenum of Cloquet. The narrower and tighter the prepuce, the better the result, as the cuts are at once converted from longitudinal into transverse wounds, and the organ at once assumes the shape and condition of a circumcised organ, without having suffered any loss of substance; three stitches or sutures in each cut (silver or catgut) adjust the cut edges; a small roller of lint and adhesive plaster, placed so as to shoulder up against the corona, completes the dressing.

Where this operation is practicable, by the thinness and narrowness of the prepuce, it has many advantages. I have repeatedly performed it on lawyers, book-keepers, clerks, and even laboring men, who have gone from the office to the courts, counting-rooms, or stores without the least resulting inconvenience or loss of time. In laborers it is better to perform the operation on a Saturday evening, which gives them a rest of thirty-six hours before going to their labor again.

The operation is comparatively painless and almost bloodless, as there need not be more than half a teaspoonful of blood lost during the operation; there is no danger of any subsequent hæmorrhage, and, with proper precautions against the occurrence of erections, from seventy-two to ninety-six hours is sufficient for a complete union; the sutures are then removed and a simple lint and adhesive-plaster dressing worn for a few days more.

In many, no more dressings are required. In many cases, with a properly adjusted dressing, that comes forward underneath so as to include the frenum, the simple dorsal slit is sufficient; but if any of the prepuce depasses the dressing underneath, it will puff and become oedematous and require frequent puncturing. To avoid it, it is better to make the Cloquet slit at once. This operation is of no value, and perfectly impracticable in a thick, pendulous prepuce. Absorption will often remove considerable preputial tissue, but where there is too much its very bulk interferes with its removal by any natural means.

Dilatation is recommended by a number of surgeons, but, I must admit, in my hands it has always proved a failure; it may be, that if the subsequent history of the cases reported as so operated upon had been carefully traced, the reports would not have been so good.

Nelaton, whose dilating instrument is generally recommended, seems, himself, to prefer some of the circumcising methods, as in the volume on *Diseases of the Genito-Urinary Organs*, in his *Surgery*, being the sixth volume of the revised edition of 1884, by Desprès, Gillettte, and Horteloup, the subject of dilatation is dismissed in two short lines.

St. Germain, of Paris, uses, as has been before observed, a two-bladed forceps, used after the manner of Nelaton, and reports good results. Dr. J. Lewis Smith agrees in his statements with Dr. St. Germain. Dr. Holgate, of New York, reports a like experience. In my own practice the prepuce has often been made *temporarily* lax and retractable, but with the usual results of the return of the contraction, with a possible thickening of the inner fold, as a result of the interference; so that only in case of any immediate demand, where the tight prepuce is producing irritation, either through pressure or adhesions, or retained sebaceous matter, do I ever resort to dilatation; always, however, even then, not as a final operation, but merely as preparatory procedure toward a future operation of a more efficient order.

In cases of timid adults, who refuse all kinds of operative interference, good results may be obtained by the use of a mild lead-wash or cold tea-baths and the introduction of flat layers of dry lint interposed between the prepuce and the glans; this has a very good effect in keeping the parts apart and dry, and may in time produce a certain amount of dilatation; but even when this is done, unless it will render the foreskin sufficiently loose to allow of its being kept finally back of the corona, it is, after all, but a temporary makeshift.

The corona should be exposed and kept clear of the preputial covering; anything short of this will not give all the good results to be desired. I have more than once performed a secondary operation on Jews, who had been imperfectly circumcised by not having the prepuce removed sufficiently, and in whom the subsequent contraction of the preputial orifice had re-covered part of the glans, and only lately visited a four-year-old boy, circumcised when eight days old, in whom the prepuce covered half of the glans, the corona acting as a tractive point from which the penile integument was being drawn forward. In this case the simple pierced-lint Maltese cross was used, with an adhesive band to hold the tails down behind and around the penis just back of the corona.

These means, although not circumcision either in a surgical or in the Hebraic religious sense, are, nevertheless, sufficient in a medical sense for all desired purposes; provided, however, that there is no resulting constriction, or a mild condition of paraphimosis, back of the corona, and that the whole of the glans is sufficiently uncovered, and that no abnormal dog-ears are left to garnish each side of the penis like an Elizabethan frill or collar; although Agnew holds that, in slitting, the practice adopted by many of rounding off the corners is mostly superfluous, as nature will do so itself in time.

The ordinary way of performing the operation by modern surgeons is by what is known as the Bumstead circumcision. It was not an invention of Bumstead, but was adopted by him in preference to all others.

The requisites are a sharp-pointed bistoury, blunt-pointed scissors, and a pair of Henry's phimosis forceps, with fine needles and fine oculists' suture silk. The penis is allowed to hang naturally and the position of the corona glandis marked on the outer skin with a pen and ink, which is to serve as a guide for the incision. The prepuce is now drawn forward until this line is brought in front of the glans and grasped between the blades of the forceps.

The prepuce is now transfixed, and, with a downward cut, that portion is severed; the knife's edge is now turned upward and the excision finished. The forceps are now removed and the integument allowed to retract; with the scissors the inner mucous fold is now split along the dorsum and trimmed off so as to leave about half an inch in front of the corona.

The parts are then brought together with the continuous suture and dressed according to the fancy of the surgeon. Care must be taken *not to bruise* the parts with the forceps, as, in such cases, sloughing of the sutured edges will be the result instead of union. I have seen this accident happen more than once, in one case being followed by a penitis that seriously complicated matters.

It has been my practice to use fine silver-wire and catgut sutures in all operations on the prepuce; they excite less suppuration as well as less irritation. In case of need, the silver can be left in longer, and they are much easier of removal than the silk; besides, they have the advantage of not cutting.

In the after-treatment the same general plan can be followed as with any amputated stump, except that it must not be forgotten that at the end of this organ dwells what has been termed the *sixth* sense, and that heat and moisture are very apt to awaken the dormant energies of the organ, even after it has undergone cruel mutilation, and even has suffered considerable loss of blood; for that reason it is best always to avoid wet or sloppy dressing, or too much ointment, as they are more apt to cause erection than to do any good.

Besides, I find water does here, as elsewhere, interfere with the deposited plastic matter, properly organizing into cicatricial tissue; so that I prefer a snug, dry dressing, which is left on for four or five days without being interfered with, and light covering, plain diet, quiet, with fifteen grains each of bromide of sodium and chloral hydrate at bed-time to insure rest and freedom from annoying erections.

Where the organ is large in its flaccid state, it is better to support it on a small oakum-stuffed pillow, made for the purpose, than to let it hang downward.

Should the stitches give way and the skin tend to retract, the plan proposed on a previous page can be followed to advantage.

In urinating, care must be taken not to soil the dressings; some patients are very careless about this if not warned. The penis should hang nearly perpendicular while in the act, and all dribbling should have ceased and the meatus and underneath be mopped dry with some soft cotton before raising the organ; nothing so irritates the parts, retards union, or is more offensive than a urine-saturated dressing.

Dr. Hue, of Rouen, uses an elastic ligature, which he introduces into the dorsal aspect of the prepuce by means of a curved needle. This he ties in front, and in three or four days it cuts its way through. Although Hue reports a large number so operated upon, the tediousness of the procedure and the swelling and oedema, as well as the active pain that must necessarily accompany the operation, will hardly recommend the ligature in preference to the incision by the knife.

Dr. Bernheim, the surgeon of the Israelitish Consistory of Paris, has operated on over eleven hundred circumcisions, besides the cases of phimosis occurring in his general practice. His opinion of the procedure of M. de Saint-Germain by dilatation is not favorable.

He has employed it in a number of cases of phimosis, at the time unfit for a more radical operation. He has, however, observed that cicatricial thickenings and recontractions are very apt to occur, and, as to the septic accidents mentioned in connection with circumcision, he has noted that they are as liable to occur in hands that are as careless and slovenly with what they do with their dilating forceps as they are with what they do with their bistouries. Dr. Bernheim prefers the circumcision forceps of Ricord, as modified by M. Mathieu. This instrument he prefers by reason of its gentler pressure, which, at the same time, is all-sufficient to properly fix the prepuce. In applying the forceps, he includes as little as possible of the lower part, keeping away as much as possible from the frenic artery. The dorsum of the inner fold he cuts with the scissors.

In children under two years of age, he simply turns this back over the free edge of the integument; in children over two years of age, he uses serres-fines. In children, he uses a piece of lint dressing steeped in a watery solution of boracic acid; in adults, he uses iodoform-gauze dressings. He finds cases unite in from three to ten days.

Dr. Bernheim warns us against using antiseptics on infants or young children, in connection with the after-dressing of circumcision. Neither phenic acid, corrosive sublimate, nor iodoform are well borne by these young subjects, and he has seen serious results follow upon as light an application as a 1/100 solution of phenic acid.

In a number of cases he reports operating with the galvano-cautery of Chardin, instead of the knife. These operations were bloodless, and cicatrization was as rapid as when the knife was used. He has in several cases operated by the dorsal incision, owing to disease of the prepuce not allowing any other operation.

In France, the Bumstead operation is known under the title of Ricord's procedure. Lisfranc, Malapert, M.

Coster, and Vidal all have operations which are not as useful as Ricord's, and have not, therefore, come into general use.

M. Sedillot condemns the dorsal incision as leaving two unsightly-looking flaps. The reverse, or inferior incision of M. Jules Cloquet is likewise not in favor with either Malgaigne or Ricord. This inferior incision or section, alongside of the frenum was first advised by Celsus. M. Cullerier contented himself with slitting the inner preputial fold, longitudinally, from its junction with the skin backward to the corona. M. Chauvin, by the aid of a complicated instrument with barbed points, drew out the mucous fold as far as possible before excising.

There is something unaccountable in the difference in results that various operations give in the hands of different surgeons. It must be that all methods are correct *with properly-chosen cases* and when properly *performed*, as well as properly looked after subsequently to the operation.

It must not be expected, however, that, in operations where the kindly assistance of nature is a thing contemplated in absorbing superfluous tissue, the case will at once give satisfaction to all. These cases must have the required time before judgment can be passed upon the merits of the operation, just as required time in cases of dilatation or in the method of M. Cullerier will often demonstrate that the benefits are but transient, and that often even cases that have been so operated upon will require a complete circumcision, *à la* Ricord or *à la* Bumstead, owing to the resulting thickening induration and overconstriction, when, if left alone, the dorsal slitting or the inferior incision of Cloquet would have previously given satisfactory results.

The final cosmetic results in the combined Cloquet and dorsal-slit operation, for instance, depend on, first, properly choosing the case. One on whom the operation is unadaptable it is useless to attempt it on, as a future circumcision or tedious and annoying re-operation of trimming would be required.

The next care is to properly cut through all constricting bands, which, like fine, tough strings, will be found to encircle the penis. These must be carefully clipped with a fine pair of strabismus scissors, as these bands do not give way, either then or afterward, of their own accord, but form the nucleus for stronger constricting bands for the future.

Then you must be sure to cut far enough back, either above or below, until you have reached where you obtain the normal and largest calibre of circumference of the penis. The adaptation of the edges of the parts and the proper application of a smooth, equal pressure, by means of the lint strap, is of the next importance; and then comes the strapping of the whole surface for about an inch and a half back of the corona, which should and must include all the tissues of the preputial part of the frenum.

A neglect or careless performance of any of the details, or the carelessness of the patient in not keeping the dressing clean, necessitating its change before the fourth day, all tend not only to interrupt the union, but to mar the future cosmetic results as well. It may be asked why all this care and trouble, and not circumcise at once? As already observed, this operation admits of the patient following his business;

whereas circumcision, on the male, will assuredly lay him up for four or five days, and perhaps ten days—something that many, be they rich or poor, cannot afford, and will not submit to.

The cosmetic condition of the penis as a copulating organ is a thing of some importance, and this should not be overlooked; for, although the particular dimension, shape, or peculiarity of the penile end never figures prominently in the complaints of women who apply for divorce—the charges being everything else under the sun—it can safely be assumed that this organ and its condition is the original, silent and unseen, as well as unconscious power behind the throne that is at the bottom of the whole business in more than one case.

Like the fable of the poor lamb that the wolf wished to devour: the real reason of his wishing to kill him was that he might eat him, the pretext set forth by the wolf that the lamb had encroached on his pasture, muddied his brook, or kept him awake by his bleating having been disproven by the lamb. Besides, it is well not to leave any distinctive or distinguishing mark, like an individual baronial crest, on the head of the organ.

To return, however, to the operative procedures, we find that Dr. Vanier finds that the operation of Cloquet by incision alongside of the frenum has the advantage of not leaving any deformity—contrary to the opinion of Ricord and Malgaigne. He, in fact, holds this procedure in such high esteem that he considers that Cloquet deserves great credit for reviving this old Celsian operation.

H. H. Smith, in his *Operative Surgery*, coincides with Vanier in his favorable opinion of this method, as he there says:

> *Frequent opportunities of testing the advantages of the plan of Cloquet having satisfied me of its value, I do not hesitate to recommend it as that best adapted to the adult, because it fully exposes the glans and leaves little or no lateral deformity, as is frequently the case with the dorsal incision,*

—an opinion that I can fully agree with, from the results of the same operation in my hands, although I have used the method even on infants.

Vanier does not approve of the dorsal incision unless it is made V-shaped, as it otherwise leaves the unsightly lateral flaps, but thinks well of the modification of Cloquet's practiced by M. Vidal de Cassis, which is performed in the following manner: The patient stands before the operator, who remains sitting; the operator seizes the prepuce on its dorsum and draws it toward him; he then introduces a narrow, sharp-pointed bistoury, with its point armed with a small waxen bullet, down alongside of the frenum until he reaches the pouched extremity of the preputial cavity at this point; the point of the bistoury is now made to transfix the waxen bullet and out through the skin, which from this point is divided from behind forward.

Vanier very sensibly suggests that the operation that is effectual, and which can be accomplished in the least number of movements or *temps*, as being the least likely to cause extensive pain and agony, should be the one preferred, and that the aim of the surgeon should be to simplify the operation by reducing the number of necessary movements.

For this reason, where an excision of considerable amount of tissue is required by the nature of the case, he prefers another operation, performed by Lallemand—that of making a dorsal transfixion and cutting off the two lateral flaps, which can all be done in three movements.

It makes but little difference as to which operation is performed on the adult, but that the subsequent dressing will exercise a good or evil influence, and greatly assist not only in the present comfort or discomfort of the patient, but in the ultimate result as well. Bearing these points in view, Charles A. Ballance, of St. Thomas's Hospital, has adopted the following procedure:

When the patient is etherized, the outline of the posterior border of the glans is marked on the skin with an aniline pencil. The skin of the prepuce is slit and removed up to the aniline line. The mucous membrane is next cut away, leaving only a free edge of about one-eighth of an inch in width. Any bleeding which occurs should be entirely arrested, and asepsis must be insured by frequent sponging with carbolic or sublimate solution. Numerous coarse-hair stitches are then inserted, so as to bring accurately together the fresh-cut edges of the skin and mucous membrane, and subsequently, after a further sponging and drying, a piece of gauze two layers of thickness, and wide enough to reach from the root of the penis nearly to the meatus, is wrapped loosely around the penis and secured by several applications of the collodion-brush. The setting of the collodion is hastened by the use of a fan, so that the air is kept in motion, and the patient should not be allowed to recover from the anæsthetic until the dressing is quite firm and hard. This dressing forms a carapace for the penis, protecting it from the bedclothes and effectually preventing the annoying and distressing erections. Mr. Ballance reports excellent results from this dressing.

—Braithwaite's *Retrospect*, July, 1888

In applying the above dressing, the shrinking incident to the drying of the collodion must not be overlooked, and the gauze layers must be loosely applied, as they would otherwise become too tight. The dressing is a very ingenious and serviceable one.

Mr. A. G. Miller, at a meeting of the Edinburgh Medico-Chirurgical Society, reported a new method of dressing after circumcision.

It consisted in first closely suturing the skin and mucous membrane by numerous catgut sutures, then painting the surface with Friar's balsam and covering it over with two or three layers of cotton wadding, on which the balsam is poured. The glans

413

*penis was left sufficiently free to allow of
water passing. The band or ring of dressing
should be at least one inch broad. The
dressing was not suitable for young infants
who were frequently wetting. In the case of
older children, they might be allowed to go
about on the second or third day, when the
dressing would be quite dry, and would not
be required to be changed or renewed.*
—Braithwaite's *Retrospect*, January, 1888

Any constricting or immovable and inelastic dressing
is subject to the same objections as plaster-of-Paris
dressings in thigh-fractures—that of being dangerous
and not expedient, unless the patient is constantly
under your eye.

Dr. Neil Macleod, in the *Edinburgh Medical Journal*
for March, 1883, advises a procedure that has always
looked favorably to me, and which I once put in
practice through the means of the ordinary ptosis
fenestrated forceps, in place of the ordinary
circumcision forceps, the sutures being introduced
through the fenestra and the prepuce cut off on the
outer side of the forceps, the thickness of the steel arm
on the outer side of the fenestra allowing of the
properly-sized border for the hold of the sutures.

Dr. Macleod places his sutures all in position
before making any incisions—a procedure which will
be found to save the patient considerable pain; as with
many the seizing and holding of the edges of the skin
and mucous membrane and the forcible pressure
exerted by the fingers or forceps while the needle is
being forced through is the most painful part of the

operation. In doing this, care must be taken to allow sufficient length to each thread to make two sutures, as well as care must be taken to properly pull out the thread in the centre between the four folds of tissue and to cut it equidistant, after the ablation of the prepuce, a blunt hook being used to fish up the threads from the preputial opening.

Erichsen favors the Jewish operation in young children, as being the easiest and safest of performance. Slitting, or the inferior or superior incision, he thought, left too much of the prepuce, which, wherever there is a tendency to phimosis, should be entirely removed,

...with a view of preserving the health and cleanliness of the parts in after life.

In the phimosis that is acquired by old men, he found dilatation with a two-bladed instrument to be sufficient, provided the indurated circle was made to yield. For the circumcision of adults he has invented an adjustable shield, something like the Jewish spatula, with which he protects the glans.

Gross (the elder) used both slitting on the dorsum and circumcision. He found neither objection nor deformity in the flaps left by the dorsal incision, as they were only temporary; in some cases, he simply followed the practice of Cullerier, of making multiple slits in the constricting and inelastic mucous membrane.

Agnew believes in circumcision in the treatment of reflex troubles. He relates a case, in the second volume of his *Surgery*, of eczema extending over the abdomen, of over a year's standing, cured in a child by circumcision; he operates by incision on the dorsum, in which he leaves nature to make away with the flaps, or he circumcises by the Bumstead method.

Van Buren and Keyes recommend both the incision on the dorsum and the operation of Ricord; where the mucous membrane alone is tight and constricted, they follow Cullerier's method of either single or multiple incisions of the inner coat. They lay great stress on the necessity of keeping the patient quietly in bed to insure rapid and complete union.

My friend, Dr. Robert J. Gregg, of San Diego, has lately operated on a number of cases, the operation being perfectly painless, the little patients submitting to it and feeling no more pain than if it were having its toe-nails trimmed, the local anæsthesia being produced by the hypodermatic injection of cocaine.

This procedure is now used to a considerable extent throughout the country, and it is a far safer and more comfortable performance than either etherizing or chloroforming, as the sudden and spasmodic filling of the lungs of young children—who will resist and hold their breath for a long time, then suddenly inhale—with anæsthetic vapor is almost unavoidable, having in two instances nearly lost two children from such an accident.

Dr. G. W. Overall, in a late *Medical Record*, which is quoted in the *Journal of the American Medical Association* of February 21, 1891, gives the description of a very good and painless method of producing this local anæsthesia; for it need hardly be said that with a nervous, irritable child the introduction of the hypodermatic needle is as formidable an operation as either slitting or the Jewish operation.

Dr. Overall is in the habit of holding a solution within the preputial cavity and then to introduce the needle in the mucous fold, having previously applied a light rubber band back of the corona, on the outer integument, so as to act like a tourniquet and limit the action of the anæsthetic effect to the prepuce.

By this procedure he avoids all pain and the operation can be performed while the child is even amusing itself, care being taken that it does not see it. Sutures that require removal should not be used, according to the Doctor, and the operation thereby becomes a perfectly painless and unalarming performance to the patient in all its details.

Peter Charles Remondino

WORKS AND AUTHORITIES QUOTED

Thèse pour le doctorat en Médecine, par J. B. B. Edmond Nogues, sur la Anatomie, Physiologie, et Pathologie du Prépuce. Paris, 1850.

Thèse à la faculté de Médecine de Strasbourg. Par J. B. A. Chauvin. Consideration sur le Phimosis et Operation de la Circoncision par un procédé nouveau. Strasbourg, 1851.

De la Circoncision chez les Egyptiens. F. Chabas. Paris, 1861.

Cause Morale de la Circoncision des Israelites. Vanier, du Havre. Paris, 1847.

La Circoncision, son importance dans la Famille et dans l'Etat. Par le Docteur Claparéde. Paris, 1861.

Dissertation sur la Circoncision, sons les rapports religieux, hygieniques, et Pathologiques. Par le Docteur Moyse Cahen. Paris, 1816.

Origine, Signification, et Histoire, de la Castration, de l'Eunuchisme, et de la Circoncision. Par le Docteur F. Bergmann de Strasbourg. Archivio per le Tradizioni Populari, vol. ii.

Darstellung der Biblichen Krankheiten. Von Dr. J. P. Trusen. Posen, 1843.

Archives Israelites de France, No. 9, 4em année, Septembre, 1843.

Bulletins de la Société d'Anthropologie de Paris. Tome x (serie iii), 3d fascicule, Juin à Octobre, 1887.

Recueil de Mémoires de Médecine, de Chirurgie, et de Pharmacie Militaires. Tome xxi (serie iii), No. 105, August, 1868.

Traité d'Hygiène, publique et privée. Michel Levy. 2d ed. Paris, 1850.

Neuroses des Organes Génito-Urinaires de l'homme. Ultzmann. Paris, 1883.

L'Hermaphrodisme, sa Nature, son Origine, ses Consequences Sociales. Par le Docteur Charles Debierre. Paris, 1886.

L'Onanisme. Tissot. Lausanne, 1787.

Traité de la nymphomanie. Dr. Bienville. Amsterdam, 1784.

La Folie Erotique. Par Prof. B. Balt. Paris, 1888.

Des Pertes Seminales Involontaires. Lallemand. Paris, 1836.

Spermatorrhoea. Lallemand and Wilson. Philadelphia, 1861.

The Philosophical Dictionary. Voltaire. London, 1765.

Oeuvres Complétes, avec notes, etc. Montesquieu. Paris, 1838.

Dictionaire d'Hygiène, publique et de salubrite. Tardieu. Paris, 1862.

Guide du Posthétomiste. Par le Docteur L. Terquem. Paris.

La Circoncision et ses suites. Par A.S. Morin. Ext. du Journal l'Excommunié, January, 1870.

La Circoncision. Par le Docteur S. Bernheim.

Circumcision. By Dr. A. B. Arnold, of Baltimore. Reprint from the *New York Medical Journal* of February 13, 1886.

Among the Cannibals. By Carl Lumholtz. New York, 1889.

Recueil de Questions proposés par une Société de savants voyageant an Arabie, Michealis. Amsterdam, 1774.

Tractatus, Alberti Bobovii, Turcarum Imp. Mohammedis IV olim Interpretis primarii, De

Turcarum Liturgia, peregrinatione Meccana, Circumcisione, Ægrotorum Visitatione, etc. Oxonii, 1690.

Le Theatre de la Turquie. Michel Le Feber. Paris, 1681.

Recherches Philosophiques sur les Americains, ou Mémoires Interessants pour servir à l'Histoire de l'Espece Humaine. Par M. de P. Augumentée par Dom Pernety. Berlin, 1774. (Also the first edition of the same work printed at Cleves in 1772.)

History of the Hebrews' Second Commonwealth. Wise. Cincinnati, 1880.

History of the Hebrew Commonwealth. Jahn. Oxford, 1840.

Jews' Letters to Voltaire. Philadelphia, 1848.

The Jewish Nation. Revised by Kidder. New York, 1850.

The Jews Under Roman Rule. By W. D. Morrison. New York, 1890.

The Story of the Jews. By James K. Hosmer. New York, 1887.

The History of the Jews. By the Rev. H. H. Milman. New York, 1843.

Early Oriental History. By John Eadie, D.D., LL.D. London, 1852.

The Bible and the Nineteenth Century. By L. T. Townsend, D.D. New York, 1889.

Legends of the Patriarchs and Prophets. By the Rev. S. Baring-Gould. New York, 1884.

The Religions of the Ancient World. By George Rawlinson, M.A. New York, 1885.

The Hermits. By the Rev. Charles Kingsley. New York, 1885.

Letters on Demonology and Witchcraft. Letters addressed to J. G. Lockhart, Esq., by Sir Walter Scott.

London, 1831.

The Philosophy of Magic, Prodigies, and Apparent Miracles. From the French of Eusebe Salvert. New York, 1855.

Atlantis, the Antediluvian World. Donnelly. New York, 1882.

Sir Thomas Browne's Works. London, 1852.

Physical Education, or the Health Laws of Nature. By Felix Oswald, M.D. New York, 1882.

The Family: an Historical and Social Study. By Thwing. Boston, 1887.

The Intellectual Development of Europe. By John W. Draper, M.D. New York, 1876.

History of European Morals. By W. E. H. Lecky, M.A. New York, 1884.

Longevity and other Biostatic Peculiarities of the Jewish Race. By John Stockton Hough. Reprinted from New York Medical Record, 1873.

Vital Statistics of the Jews. By Dr. John S. Billings, in North American Review for January, 1891.

On Regimen and Longevity. By John Bell, M.D. New York, 1842.

Diseases of Modern Life. By B. W. Richardson, M.D. New York, 1876.

Cyclopedia of Biblical, Theological, and Ecclesiastical Literature. By McClintock and Strong. New York, 1886.

Early History of Mankind. Tylor. London, 1870.

Dictionaire des Sciences Médicales. 60-vol. edition. Paris, 1816.

British and Foreign Medico-Chirurgical Review, vols. for 1846, 1854, 1856, 1858, 1863, 1868, and 1869. London.

Braithwaite's Retrospect of Medicine and Surgery.

The Chinese. John Francis Davis, Esq., F.R.S. London, 1851.

Massachusetts State Board of Health Report for 1873.

On Diseases of Children. Stewart. New York, 1844.

Diseases of Children. West. Philadelphia.

Lectures on Diseases of Children. Henoch. New York, 1882.

Women's and Children's Diseases. Dillnberger. Philadelphia, 1871.

Male Impotence. Hammond. New York, 1883.

Genito-Urinary Diseases. Otis. New York, 1883.

Urinary and Renal Diseases. Roberts. Philadelphia, 1885.

Urinary and Renal Disorders. Beale.

Renal and Urinary Organs. Black. Philadelphia, 1872.

Gout in its Protean Aspects. Fothergill. Detroit, 1883.

Venereal Diseases. Bumstead and Taylor. Philadelphia, 1883.

Traité sur les Maladies des Organes Génito-Urinaires. Civiale. Paris, 1850.

Pathologic Chirurgicale, tome vi. Nelaton. Paris, 1884.

Pathologie Externe, tome v. Vidal (de Cassis). Paris, 1846.

Guy's Hospital Reports, 3d series, vol. xvii. London, 1872.

Transactions of the Ninth International Medical Congress, vol iii. Washington, 1887.

American Journal of Obstetrics for January, 1882.

On the Reproductive Organs. Acton. Philadelphia, 1883.

Operative Surgery. Smith. Philadelphia, 1852.

Operative Surgery. Stephen Smith. Philadelphia, 1887.

System of Surgery. Gross. Philadelphia, 1859.

Principles and Practice of Surgery. Agnew. Philadelphia,

1881.

International Encyclopedia of Surgery. Ashhurst. Philadelphia, 1886.

Science and Art of Surgery. Erichsen. Philadelphia, 1869.

Diseases of the Kidneys. Ralfe. Philadelphia, 1885.

The Clinic. Cincinnati, 1872.

American Journal of the Medical Sciences for July, 1872; also vol. lx.

New York Medical Journal, vols. xvi, xix, xxvi.

Occidental Medical Times. Sacramento, October, 1890.

London Lancet, 1875.

Distribution Geographique de la Phthisie Pulmonaire. Lancereaux. Paris, 1877.

Annual Report of the Bureau of Ethnology. J. W. Powell. Washington, 1884.

Western Journal of Medicine and Surgery. Louisville, 1846.

Native Races of the Pacific Coast. Bancroft. San Francisco, 1875.

Encyclopedia Britannica, 9th edition.

Classical Dictionary. Lempriere. New York, 1847.

Commentary on the Bible. Clark.

Satellite for February, 1889, and January, 1891. Philadelphia.

Pedigree of Diseases. Hutchinson.

Medical Inquiries. Rush. Philadelphia.

Half-Yearly Abstract of the Medical Sciences, vols. xii and lx, Philadelphia.

Cincinnati Lancet and Observer, vol. xvi.

Statistics and Climate of Consumption. Millard.

Traité des Maladies Chirurgicales, vol. x. Baron Boyer. Paris, 1825.

Dictionary of Medicine. Quain. New York, 1884.

INDEX

Publishers Note

In the interest of saving paper, I deleted the Index section of this book. Here's the thought process: if a reader or researcher wants to search the text for keywords of interest, this should be done by taking advantage of technology and using a search tool in the eBook version. Please note: all purchasers of the printed book can get a free eBook version from Stairway Press...shoot us an email and we'll send it along.

—KLC

www.ingramcontent.com/pod-product-compliance
Lightning Source LLC
Chambersburg PA
CBHW021351090426
42742CB00009B/808